# Orthodontics Picture Tes

*Senior commissioning editor:* Mary Seager
*Development editor:* Caroline Savage
*Production controller:* Anthony Read
*Desk editor:* Angela Davies
*Cover designer:* Alan Studholme

# Orthodontics Picture Test Atlas

**Claire Nightingale**
MSc BDS (Hons.) FDS RCS (Eng.) MOrthRCS (Edin.)
*Senior Registrar, Eastman Dental Hospital, London, and*
*Queen Mary's University Hospital, Roehampton, UK*

and

**Jonathan Sandy**
PhD MOrth FDS FMedSci
*Professor of Orthodontics, Bristol Dental School, University of Bristol, UK*

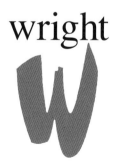
wright

OXFORD  AUCKLAND  BOSTON  JOHANNESBURG  MELBOURNE  NEW DELHI

Wright
An imprint of Butterworth-Heinemann
Linacre House, Jordan Hill, Oxford OX2 8DP
225 Wildwood Avenue, Woburn, MA 01801-2041
A division of Reed Educational and Professional Publishing Ltd

 A member of the Reed Elsevier plc group

First published 2001

**British Library Cataloguing in Publication Data**
Nightingale, Claire
 Orthodontics picture test atlas
 1 Orthodontics   2 Orthodontics – Diagnosis
 I Title  II Sandy, Jonathan
 617.6'43

**Library of Congress Cataloguing in Publication Data**
Nightingale, Claire.
 Orthodontics picture test atlas / Claire Nightingale and Jonathan Sandy.
 p. ; cm.
 Includes bibliographical references and index.
 1. Malocclusion–Examinations, questions, etc   2. Malocclusion–Atlases
 3 Orthodontic appliances–Examinations, questions, etc.   4 Orthodontic
 appliances–Atlases   5 Occlusion (Dentistry)–Examinations, questions,
 etc.   6 Occlusion (Dentistry)–Atlases   7 Orthodontics–Examinations,
 questions, etc.   8 Orthodontics–Atlases   I. Sandy, Jonathan   II Title.
 [DNLM: 1. Malocclusion–diagnosis–Examination Questions   2
 Malocclusion–therapy–Examination Questions   3. Orthodontic
 Appliances–Examination Questions   WU 18.2 N688o 2000]
 RK523 .N54
 617.6'43'0076–dc21                                        00–056440

ISBN 0 7236 1072 X

Composition by Scribe Design, Gillingham, Kent
Printed in Great Britain at the University Press, Cambridge

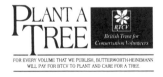

# Contents

# Foreword

In the past few years several excellent new undergraduate orthodontic textbooks have appeared. These all follow the same general format and aim to cover the principles of aetiology, case assessment and treatment planning which the student will need to know. Just as important is the need for the new graduate to recognise developing occlusal problems promptly, so that these children can be referred for effective specialist treatment. This new volume by Claire Nightingale and Jonathan Sandy is to be welcomed, since it has been designed to allow students and new graduates to test and improve their knowledge in the recognition of everyday occlusal anomalies. The problem-based approach and the authors' clear layout and description are bound to be both popular and effective. They will help ensure that children and parents receive informed advice and prompt referral from the next generation of general dental practitioners.

Professor Chris Stephens
Bristol, September 2000

# Preface

This book is the result of collaboration between former pupil (CN) and teacher (JRS). The first postgraduate course in orthodontics (1993–1996) at Bristol Dental School was a steep learning curve for both authors: for Claire, who established orthodontic understanding from a position of ignorance, and for Jonathan, who learnt to teach a group from first principles. Experience in teaching both undergraduate and postgraduate dental students, and working with general dental practitioners, suggested a need for an illustrated question and answer book, where the basics are explained with the help of a visual aid. This book is intended to supplement the undergraduate dental curriculum and the questions should be attempted when the fundamental knowledge has been gained. Some of the answers are written in more depth than would be expected from an undergraduate, in the hope that this will offer greater clarity of understanding and will benefit also the postgraduate orthodontist and the interested general dental practitioner.

We have not intended to teach clinical technique, as we consider this to be the realm of a structured specialist training programme. However, we hope that undergraduates would be confident enough to treat simple problems with removable appliances, such as pushing a tooth over the bite. Therefore removable appliances have been considered in some detail. We hope that the chapters on examination and diagnosis and on treatment planning will help the general dental practitioner identify orthodontic problems at a suitable stage in occlusal development and will enhance dialogue with the specialist orthodontic practitioner. The remaining chapters will aid discussion with patients and parents and help to identify the problems that can arise during orthodontic treatment.

In common with other books of this nature, we have not supported our answers with references. We support the principle of evidence-based dentistry but believe there are many more appropriate texts which provide this. Above all, we hope that we have written a book that will be both interesting and enlightening to those who are trying to increase their understanding of this specialist clinical area.

Claire Nightingale
Jonathan Sandy
England, September 2000

# Acknowledgements

We are very grateful for the helpful comments made by Dr Tony Ireland, Mrs Dorothy Nattrass, Mr Ed Payne, Mrs Alicia Thompson and Mrs Ranji Uthayashankar during the preparation of this book. We would like to thank Bristol Dental Hospital; the Eastman Dental Hospital; the orthodontic departments of: the Royal United Hospital, Bath; Southmead Hospital, Bristol; and the Queen Mary's University Hospital, Roehampton, for the use of photographs of patients treated within these units. We are also grateful for the images supplied by Mr Allan Jones (Figure 5.2) and Dr Yang Soon Chia (Figure 5.4) and would like to thank the patients who consented to appear in this book. Finally, we thank Miss Jane Western for her cheerful secretarial assistance and Stuart Nightingale and Jackie Sandy for their endless support and understanding throughout the production of this book.

# Questions

# Ideal occlusion

## Question 1.1

a) How would you classify this incisor relationship?
b) What are the other occlusal features you can see?
c) What are Andrew's six keys to normal static occlusion?
d) What is the difference between an Angle's and an Andrew's class I molar relationship?

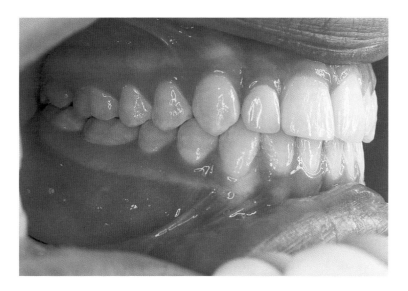

# Question 1.2

a) What do you see here?
b) What is the name given to this type of functional occlusal relationship?
c) What are the features of this type of dynamic occlusion?
d) What is the other main type of dynamic occlusion?

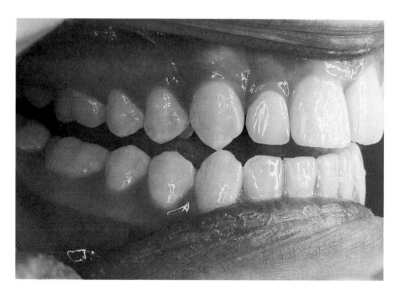

# Examination and diagnosis

## Question 2.1

a) What would you assess during an extraoral orthodontic examination?
b) What would you assess during an intraoral orthodontic examination?
c) What adjunctive procedures would aid diagnosis?

# Question 2.2

a)  What is the anteroposterior skeletal relationship shown here?
b)  How are the maxilla and mandible related in this type of skeletal relationship?
c)  The cephalometric value ANB in the Eastman Analysis indicates anteroposterior skeletal relationship. What is the likely value of the angle ANB in the skeletal relationship shown?
d)  It is important to assess vertical skeletal pattern as well as the anteroposterior skeletal relationship. What is a normal vertical skeletal relationship and what is the normal value of the Frankfort-mandibular planes angle?

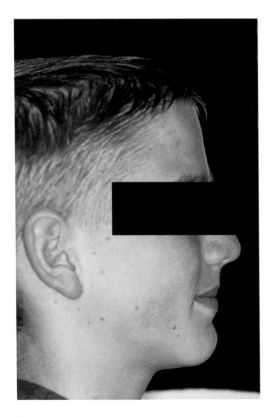

# Question 2.3

a) Classify this malocclusion.
b) What methods are used to relieve crowding?
c) Which feature of this malocclusion suggests that this patient needs treatment with fixed appliances?

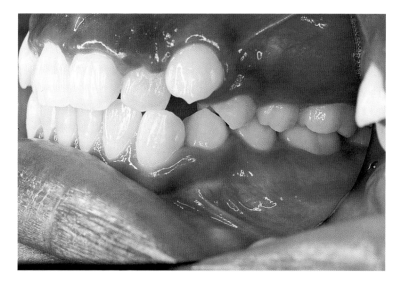

# Question 2.4

a) What type of malocclusion is seen here in this 11 year old girl?
b) A number of aetiological factors can result in this malocclusion. What factors would you consider?
c) What treatment options would you consider?

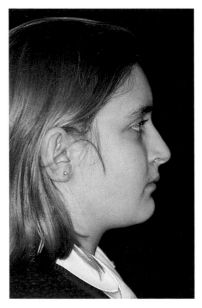

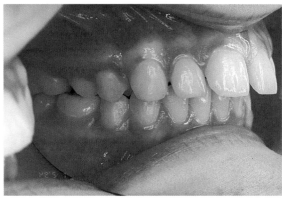

# Question 2.5

a) Assess the extraoral features seen here.
b) Describe and classify the malocclusion.
c) This case is amenable to orthodontic correction. Which dimension in particular must be carefully controlled during treatment and why?
d) Will the result be stable after orthodontic treatment?
e) Why does she have gingivitis?

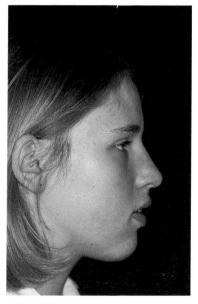

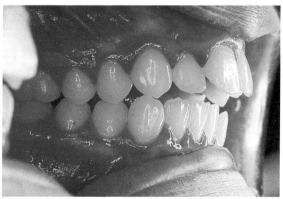

# Question 2.6

a) Assess the extraoral features of this patient.
b) Describe her occlusion and account for the buccal segment asymmetry.
c) The upper lateral incisors are slightly small. What effect will this have on occlusion after treatment?
d) She is 18 years old, and greatly dislikes her 'gummy' smile and increased overjet. What treatment options would you discuss with her?

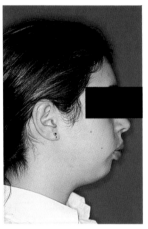
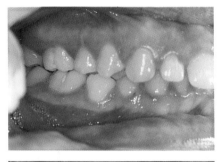
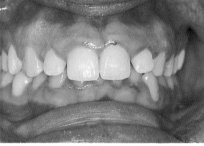
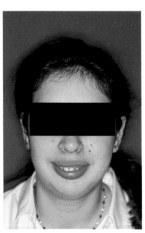
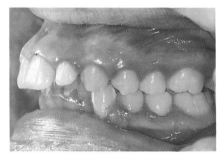

# Question 2.7

a) What dental and skeletal relationship do you see here?
b) Describe the key features of the soft tissue profile.
c) What is the principal cause of his increased overjet (15 mm) and what factors will influence post-treatment stability once the overjet has been reduced?

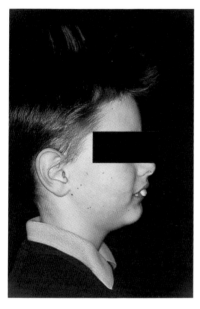

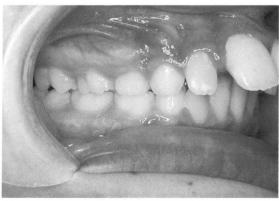

# Question 2.8

a) Describe the skeletal relationship shown here.
b) What value of the angle ANB is typical of this type of antero-posterior skeletal relationship?
c) The patient has a class II division 2 type incisor relationship. What are the skeletal and soft tissue features commonly seen with this malocclusion?
d) Which of her facial features masks the skeletal relationship?

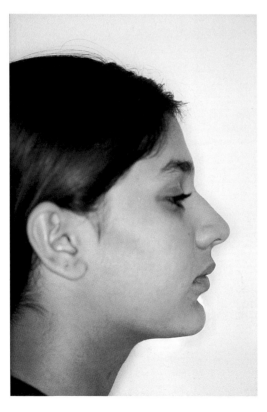

# Question 2.9

a) Describe the buccal segment and incisor relationships.
b) Classify and define this malocclusion.
c) What are the dental features of this type of malocclusion?
d) Which principal feature of this malocclusion must be corrected to give the best chance of stability?
e) What is the cause of the upper incisor inclination?

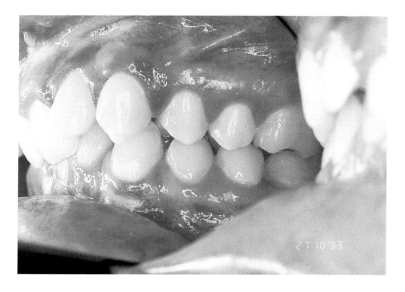

# Question 2.10

a) Assess the extraoral features of this 14 year old boy.
b) Describe and classify his malocclusion.
c) This malocclusion is amenable to orthodontic correction. What are the aims of treatment?
d) What principal factor would limit the success of orthodontic treatment?

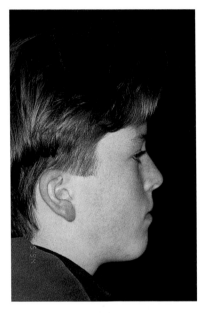

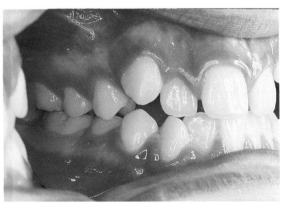

# Question 2.11

a)  What do these photographs demonstrate and what is the clinical significance?
b)  What are the skeletal features commonly seen in people with this malocclusion?
c)  Why is the buccal segment relationship class I, but the incisor relationship class III?

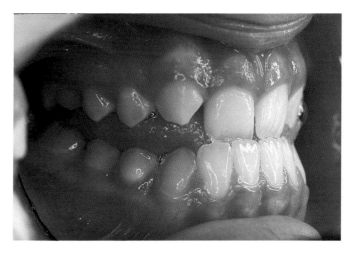

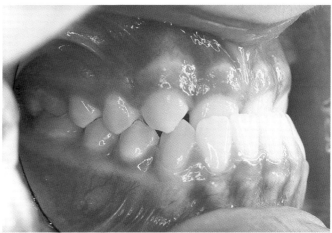

# Question 2.12

a) What type of skeletal relationship is this?
b) What value of the angle ANB is typical of this type of skeletal relationship?
c) How is the maxilla related to the mandible anteroposteriorly?
d) What is the cause of the anterior open bite?
e) Is this case likely to be amenable to orthodontic correction?

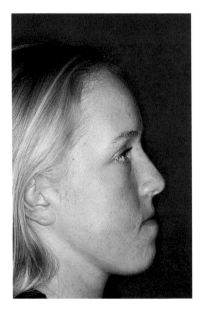

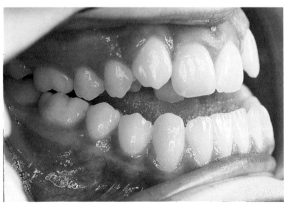

# Question 2.13

a) What skeletal relationship do you see here?
b) Describe the buccal segment relationship and the incisor relationship.
c) The incisor relationship and facial profile suggest that the malocclusion is not as severe as the buccal segment relationship demonstrates. Explain this apparent anomaly.

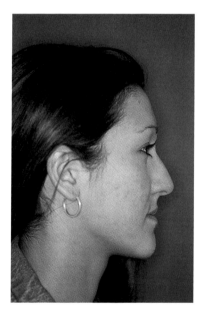

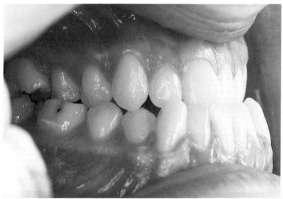

# Question 2.14

a) What do you see here?
b) Why is growth potential important in assessing this problem?
c) Why is it important to detect mandibular displacements on closure?
d) How would you manage a lateral mandibular displacement in a child in the mixed dentition?

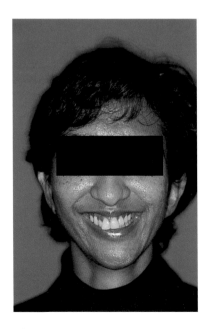

# Question 2.15

a) What type of malocclusion is shown here?
b) In which ethnic groups is this problem more common?
c) What is the aetiology of this malocclusion?
d) What are the common motives for having orthodontic treatment?
e) What factors influence the long-term stability of treated cases?

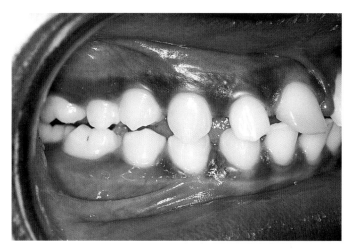

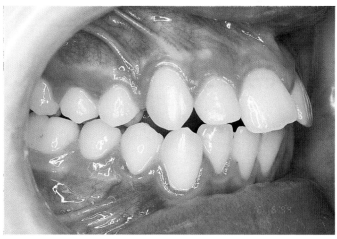

# Question 2.16

a)  When should the upper permanent canines i) be palpable and
    ii) erupt?
b)  What feature of this maxillary arch causes concern?
c)  What investigations should you carry out?
d)  What treatment options would you consider?

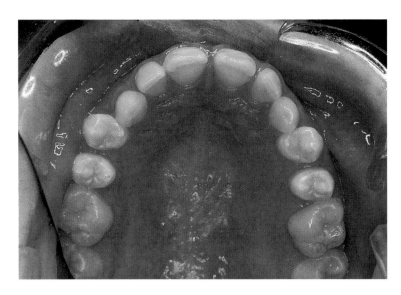

# Question 2.17

a) What has happened here?
b) What is the incidence of this problem?
c) Is this more common in males or in females?
d) What factors are associated with this condition?
e) What are the risks associated with this problem?

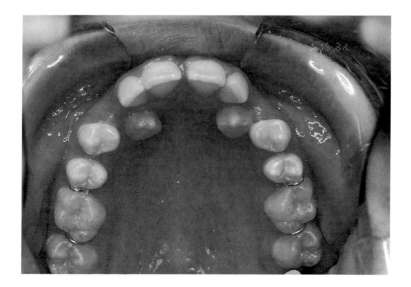

# Question 2.18

a) What do you see here?
b) What are the possible causes?
c) What will need to be monitored carefully during orthodontic treatment?

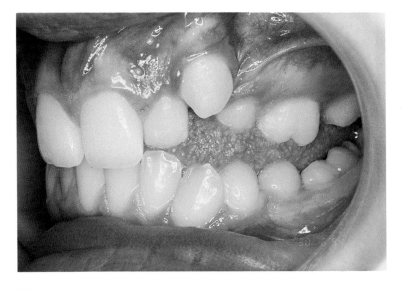

# Question 2.19

a) What do you see here?
b) What is the likely cause of this malocclusion?
c) What are the skeletal and dental features associated with this problem long term?
d) How would you manage this case in the first instance?

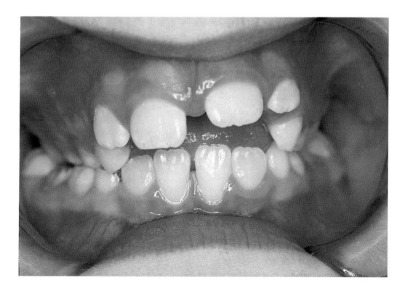

# Question 2.20

a) Describe what you see here.
b) Is this a significant problem?
c) How would you manage this?
d) Design the appliance you would use to correct this problem.
   Teeth present are:

| 6EDC21 | 12CDE6 |
|--------|--------|
| 6EDC21 | 12CDE6 |

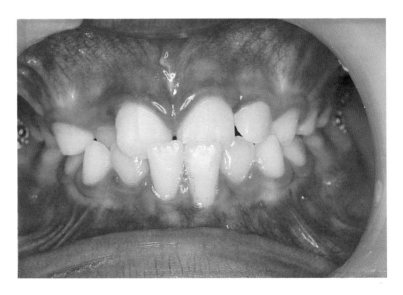

# Question 2.21

a) What has happened here?
b) How common is this problem and is it more frequent in females or in males?
c) What factors would influence treatment?
d) What are the aetiological factors contributing to this problem?

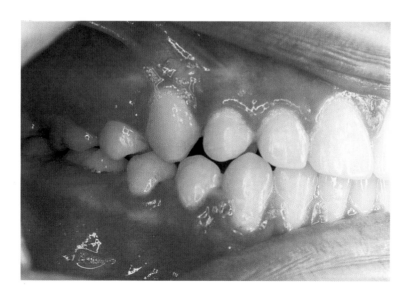

# Question 2.22

a) What can you see here?
b) How should the space be maintained before orthodontic treatment?
c) How can aesthetics be managed during orthodontic treatment?
d) What options would you discuss with the patient for restorative management after orthodontic treatment?

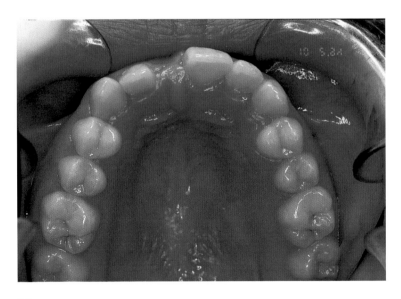

# Question 2.23

a) Describe what you see here.
b) What has happened to the deciduous molars?
c) What is the prognosis for the permanent dentition?
d) What are the possible causes of the anterior open bite?

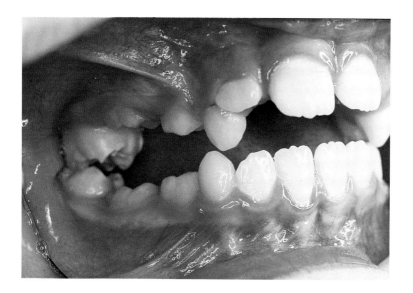

# Question 2.24

a) Describe what you see here.
b) How would you investigate this problem?
c) What treatment options would you consider?
d) What aetiological factors may have caused this problem?

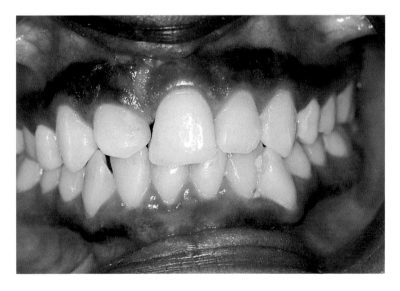

# Question 2.25

a) What condition does this radiograph demonstrate?
b) This patient is 12 years old. Which teeth are missing?
c) List the most commonly missing teeth in the Caucasian population and give the incidence rate for each.
d) What is the most commonly missing tooth in the Japanese population?
e) Name three syndromes associated with missing teeth.

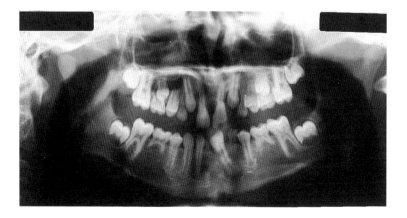

# Question 2.26

a) What problem is shown here?
b) What is the incidence of this problem?
c) What treatment options would you discuss?
d) How can the teeth adjacent to the central incisors be modified for better aesthetics?

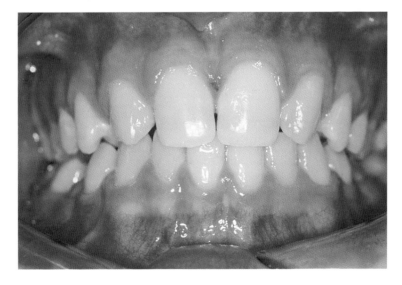

# Question 2.27

a) What do you see here?
b) What is the cause of this problem?
c) How should this be managed?

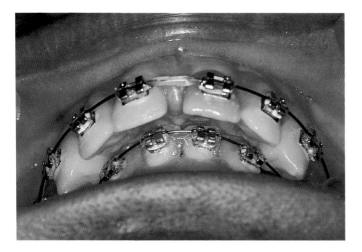

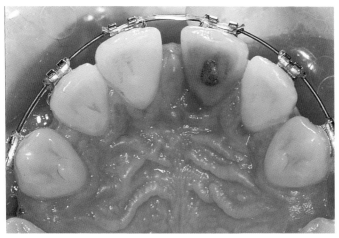

# 3 Treatment planning

## Question 3.1

a) The aims of orthodontic treatment are particular for each patient, depending on the presenting features of the malocclusion. However, there are some general aims of treatment. What are these?

b) What is the importance of assessing the skeletal relationship in all three planes?

c) What is the relationship between the vertical dimension and the decision to extract teeth?

# Question 3.2

a) Why is growth potential significant in the assessment of skeletal relationship?
b) Which treatment aims are most helped by favourable growth?
c) When is the pubertal growth spurt in i) girls and ii) boys?
d) What is a backward mandibular growth rotation and what is its importance to:
   i)    the correction of class II skeletal relationship?
   ii)   overbite management?
   iii)  treatment mechanics?

# Question 3.3

a) What is the importance of establishing a normal overbite?
b) What is the relationship between the vertical skeletal dimension and overbite?
c) How does the overbite affect overjet management?
d) Why is overbite reduction easier in a growing patient than in an adult?
e) List methods of overbite reduction.

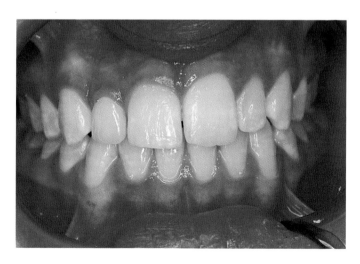

# Question 3.4

a) How many millimetres of crowding would be described as i) mild, ii) moderate and iii) severe? How crowded is this arch?

b) A premolar width is approximately 7 mm and this is described as one unit. What buccal segment relationship will result at the end of orthodontic treatment following the removal of: i) one unit in each quadrant, ii) two units in the lower arch only and iii) two units in the upper arch only, in a patient with a full complement of permanent teeth and a class I skeletal relationship?

c) What factors would you take into account when planning extractions?

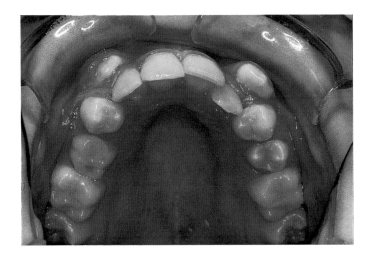

# Question 3.5

a) Following orthodontic diagnosis and establishment of treatment aims, what is the starting point for treatment planning?
b) Which dimensions should not be altered during treatment?

# Question 3.6

a) At what stage of dental development is this child?
b) What is the most important diagnosis at this stage?
c) What would be the likely effect of early unilateral loss of a deciduous canine on the developing dentition?
d) What would be the likely effect of early unilateral loss of a deciduous second molar on the developing dentition?
e) What interceptive measures would you consider to manage a maxillary permanent canine that appears to be palatally positioned?

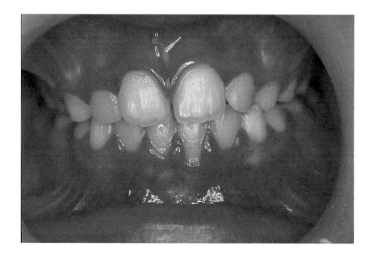

# Question 3.7

a) What is balancing extraction and when would you consider this?

b) What is compensating extraction and when would you recommend it?

c) When would you consider providing a space maintainer?

# Question 3.8

a) This is a lateral cephalometric radiograph. How should the patient be positioned when it is taken?
b) Why are these radiographs taken?
c) What steps should be taken to produce an optimum image?

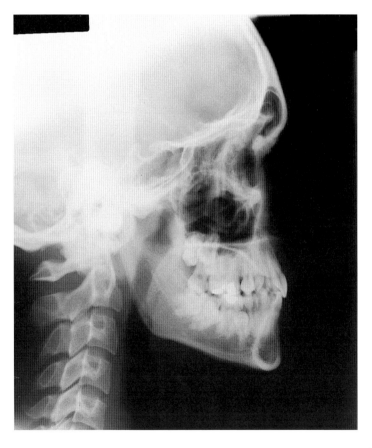

# Question 3.9

This is a tracing of a cephalometric radiograph of patient SF. The following values were obtained from the tracing:

| | |
|---|---|
| SNA | = 81.5° |
| SNB | = 93.5° |
| ANB | = −12° |
| Maxillary mandibular plane | = 15° |
| Overjet | = −2 mm |
| Upper incisors to maxillary plane | = 133° |
| Lower incisors to mandibular plane | = 80° |

a) Describe the skeletal relationship both vertically and anterio-posteriorly.
b) Compare the incisor angulations to normal Caucasian values and account for the differences.
c) Describe the overjet. Is this what you would expect to find in a patient with this skeletal relationship?
d) Is the maxilla normally positioned?
e) Will this patient's malocclusion be manageable by orthodontics alone?

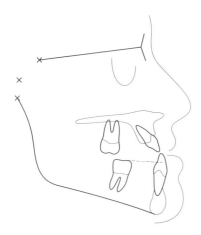

# Question 3.10

The following values were obtained from a tracing of a lateral cephalometric radiograph of patient KS:

| | |
|---|---|
| SN | = 81.5° |
| SNB | = 75.5° |
| ANB | = 6° |
| Maxillary mandibular plane | = 24.5° |
| Overjet | = 6 mm |
| Upper incisors to maxillary plane | = 99° |
| Lower incisors to mandibular plane | = 98° |

a)  Describe the incisor relationship.
b)  Which jaw is likely to be the cause of the skeletal discrepancy and why?
c)  Comment on the inclination of the incisors and describe what effect this has had on the overjet.

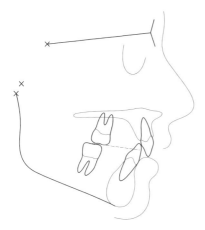

# Question 3.11

The IOTN and PAR Indices are well-established in orthodontics.
a)  What do the acronyms stand for?
b)  What is the difference between them?
c)  How is the IOTN further divided?

# Pathology

## Question 4.1

a) What is this?
b) How frequently does it occur?
c) What causes it?
d) Describe the mechanism and timing of palatal shelf closure.

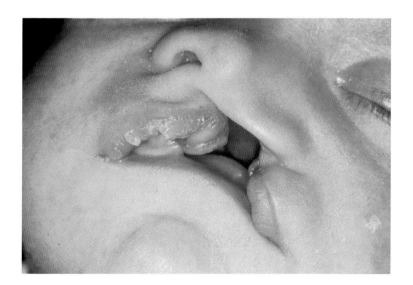

# Question 4.2

a) Unilateral cleft lip and palate comprise the most common form of facial clefting. What are the other expressions of clefting in humans?

b) This photograph demonstrates a cleft lip repair. What is the typical surgical management of repair of clefts?

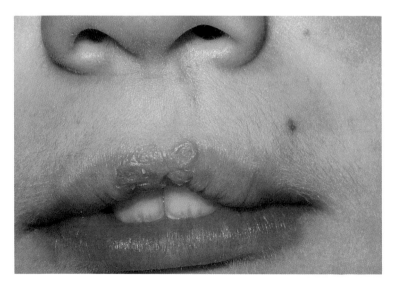

# Question 4.3

a)  How is the dentition affected in patients with clefting?
b)  What are the major issues of concern in the dental manage-
    ment of these patients?

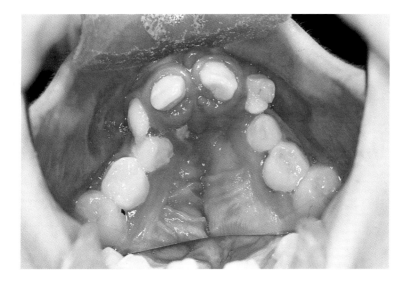

# Question 4.4

a) What soft tissue abnormality is seen here?
b) What effect can it have on the dentition?
c) What treatment should be considered?
d) What physical sign is a guide to prescribing surgery?

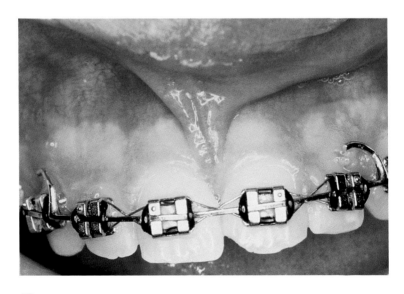

# Question 4.5

a) What is this?
b) Is this a common appearance?
c) What is the incidence of this problem?
d) What other problems can arise?

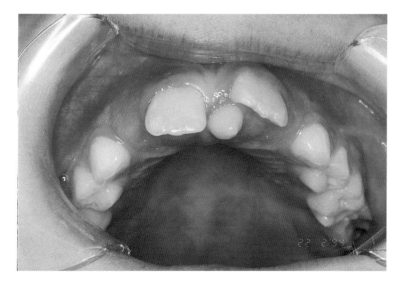

# Question 4.6

a) What abnormality in eruption is seen here?
b) How should this be managed?
c) What are the common causes of this problem?

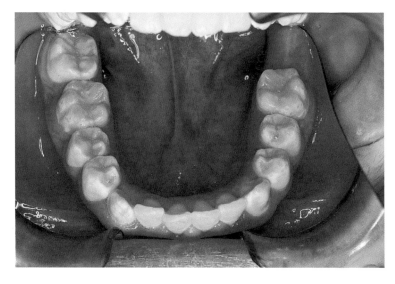

# Question 4.7

This is a histological section of a tooth with periodontal ligament and bone.
a) Describe the activity at the bone/periodontal interface.
b) How vascular is the periodontal ligament?
c) In which direction is the tooth moving?

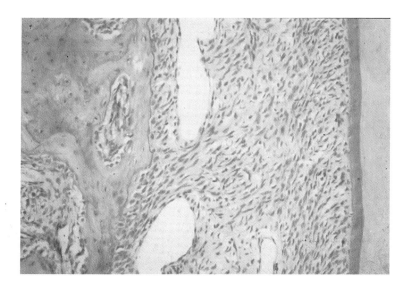

# Question 4.8

This is a compressed periodontal ligament.
a) Describe the appearance.
b) What is likely to happen once the force has been removed?
c) Why is this condition undesirable during orthodontic tooth movement?

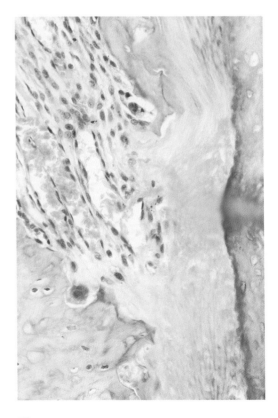

# Question 4.9

This is a histological section demonstrating tooth movement.
a) Describe the bone/periodontal interface.
b) In which direction is the tooth moving?
c) What is the likely origin of the large multi-nucleate cells (osteoclasts)?

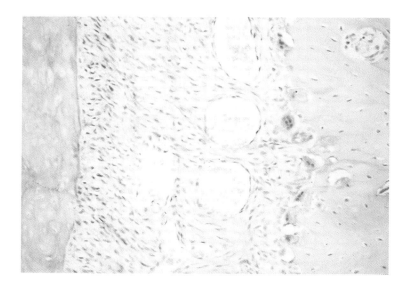

# Removable appliances

## Question 5.1

a) What is the fundamental difference between tooth movement achieved with removable and with fixed appliances?
b) What controls the force delivered by removable appliances and what is considered to be the optimal force?
c) What are removable appliances used for in current orthodontic practice?
d) What are the advantages and disadvantages of removable appliances as compared with fixed appliances?

# Question 5.2

a)  It is useful to use the acronym ARAB as a memory aid when designing removable appliances. What does this stand for?

b)  Design an appliance to push the upper incisors over the bite. Teeth present are:

| 6EDC1 | 12CDE6 |
|-------|--------|
| 6EDC21 | 12CDE6 |

c)  Is retention necessary after treatment?

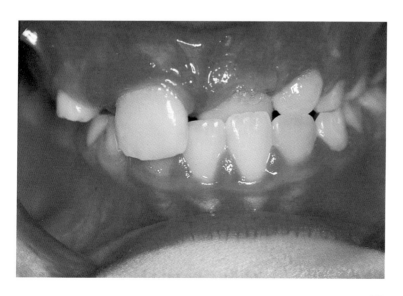

# Question 5.3

a) What is the anterior component of this appliance called and what is it used for?
b) How is it activated and how is the amount of activation measured?
c) What alternative components attached to a removable appliance could be used instead?
d) What should be considered when fitting the appliance?

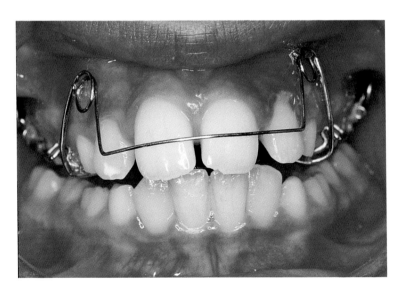

# Question 5.4

a)  What is this appliance being used for?
b)  Is the canine palatal finger spring correctly activated?
c)  What other spring design could you use instead?
d)  Draw two possible designs for this appliance.
e)  What must be considered when the appliance is fitted?

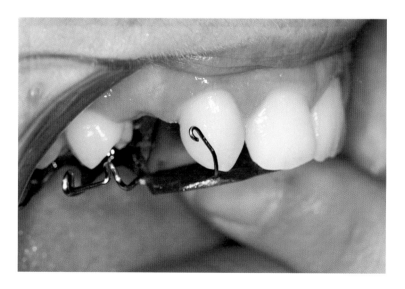

# Question 5.5

a) What are the two functions of this appliance?
b) How often should the screw be turned and how much activation does this achieve?
c) What is the disadvantage of this method of expansion?
d) What other methods of upper arch expansion do you know?
e) What is the function of the posterior bite capping and of what should the patient and parent be warned?
f) How are the T springs activated and what alternative springs could be used?
g) Which feature of the malocclusion will be the most prone to relapse?
h) Draw a design for this appliance.

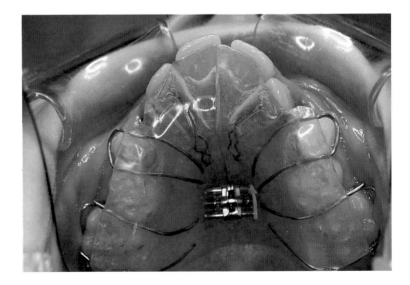

# Question 5.6

a) What is the purpose of this appliance?
b) What are the problems with its use?
c) What is the purpose of the posterior capping?
d) Why are tubes soldered to the bridge of the Adams cribs?

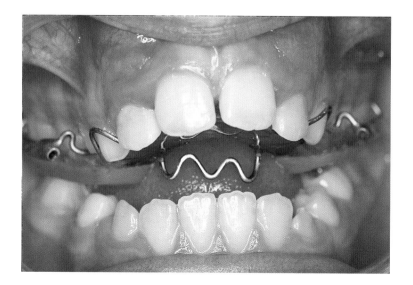

# Question 5.7

a) Draw designs for the following upper removable appliances (URA). Assume all permanent teeth excluding third molars are present.
- i) An appliance designed to distalize the upper first molars in conjunction with headgear attached to molar band
- ii) A clip overbite plane to be used with fixed appliances
- iii) A space maintainer for a missing upper left central incisor
- iv) An appliance designed to achieve unilateral crossbite correction of the upper right buccal segment
- v) An appliance designed to distalize the upper left buccal segment.

b) All appliances used to distalize teeth may cause one common problem. What is this, and how can it be monitored and controlled?

# Functional appliances

## Question 6.1

a) What appliance is this?
b) How is it retained?
c) Which malocclusion is particularly suited to treatment with this type of appliance and why?
d) What are its limitations?

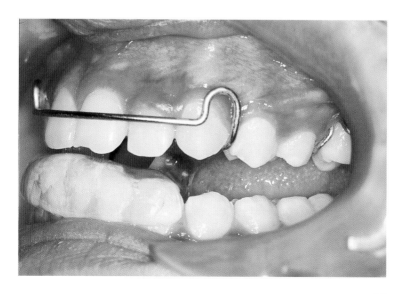

# Question 6.2

a) What type of appliance is this?
b) When would you use it?
c) How does it work?
d) What is the advantage of this appliance over other functional appliances?
e) How would you attach headgear if required? Why is addition of extraoral traction (EOT) an advantage?

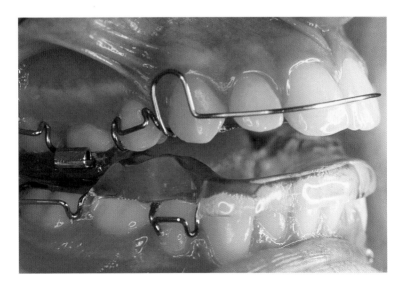

# Question 6.3

a) What type of appliance is this?
b) What is its country of origin?
c) How does it work?
d) Describe possible alternative treatment options for the management of a developing class III malocclusion.

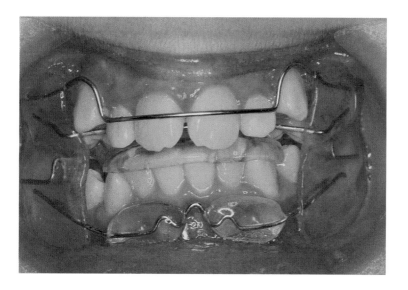

# Fixed appliances

## Question 7.1

a) What appliance is this?
b) How can you distinguish between the straightwire and standard edgewise appliances?
c) What are the advantages of straightwire appliances over standard edgewise appliances?
d) What components are used for a fixed appliance and how are they attached?
e) What type of elastic wear is this?

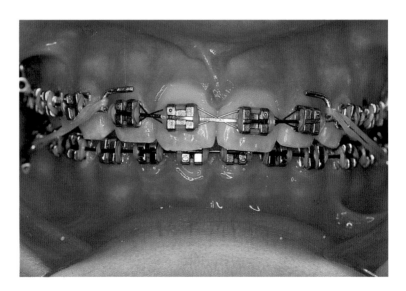

## Question 7.2

a) What type of fixed appliance is this and which technique is its predecessor?
b) How does its mode of action differ from that of the straightwire appliance?
c) What should be achieved in each stage of treatment?
d) What is the mechanical driving force used in this system and how are its unwanted side-effects controlled?

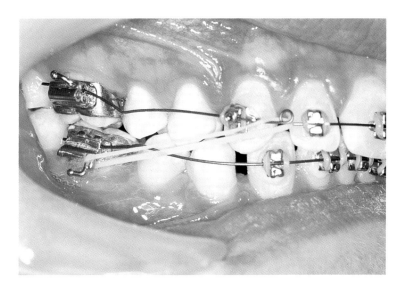

# Question 7.3

a) What can be seen here?
b) What are the advantages and disadvantages of this type of bracket?
c) How are the disadvantages being overcome?

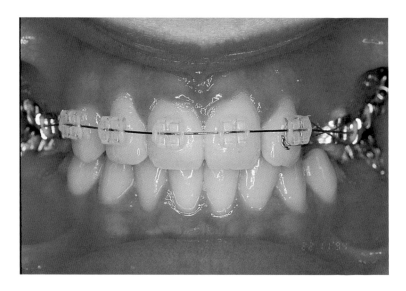

# Question 7.4

a) What type of appliance is this?
b) What is it used for?
c) What is the normal amount of activation?
d) What problems might be expected?
e) What alternative appliances could be used?

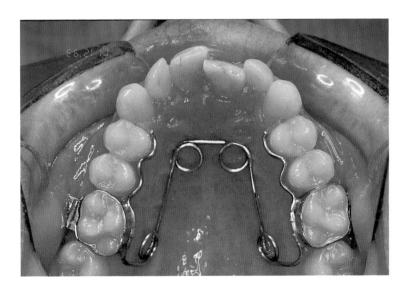

# Question 7.5

a) What is this appliance called?
b) How often should the screw be turned and when should the patient be reviewed after fitting?
c) Of what should the patient be warned?
d) What is the difference between the expansion achieved using this appliance and that obtained with other appliances?

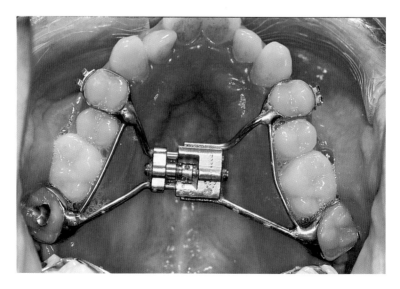

# Question 7.6

a) What are the desirable properties of an orthodontic wire?
b) What effect does increasing the cross-section of a wire have on its properties?
c) What effect does increasing the length of a wire have on the forces being applied to teeth?

# Question 7.7

a) Why is this wire being cooled with a refrigerant on a cotton wool pellet?

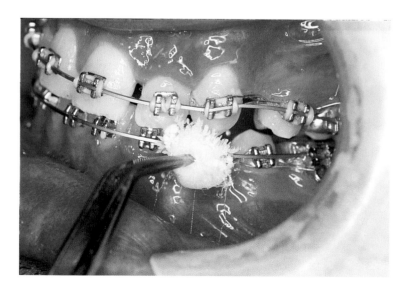

## Question 8.1

a) What appliance is this?
b) What is its function and when is its use indicated?
c) Describe the clinical steps in its fabrication.
d) What problem might arise during transit to the laboratory?
e) What alternative appliance might be considered?

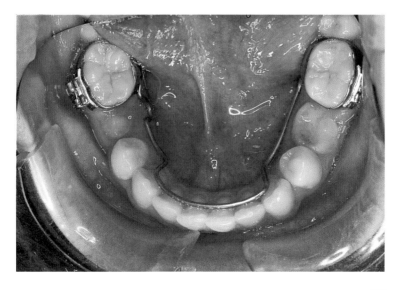

# Question 8.2

a) What type of appliance is this?
b) When would you use it?
c) What are the component parts of the system shown here?
d) What force would you apply and for how long?
e) What precautions must be taken if this appliance is used?

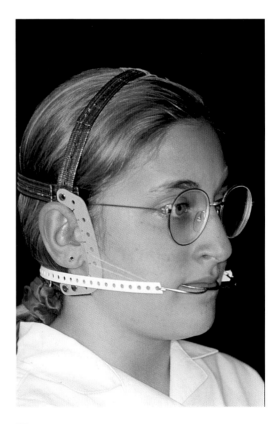

# Question 8.3

a) Describe this buccal segment relationship.
b) Give a possible explanation for this appearance.
c) The patient wishes to have comprehensive orthodontic treatment with full reduction of his 8 mm overjet. He has a class I skeletal relationship of normal vertical dimension with competent lips. What options are available for him?

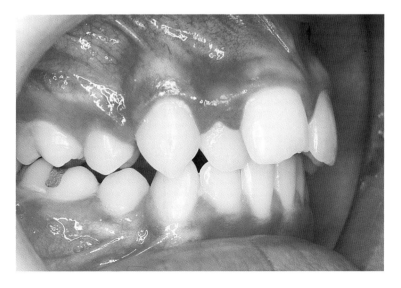

# Question 8.4

a) What appliance is this?
b) What is it used for?
c) What are the problems which patients may experience in wearing the appliance?
d) To what is it attached intraorally?

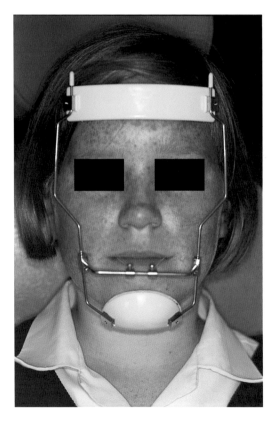

## Question 9.1

a)  What has happened during treatment?
b)  What has caused this?
c)  Is this a common problem?
d)  How might it be avoided during treatment?
e)  What remedies are available?

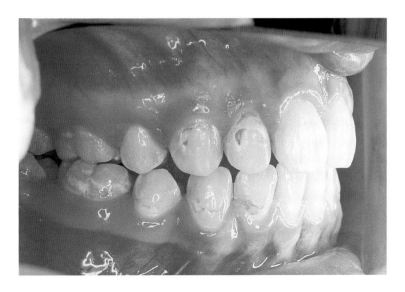

# Question 9.2

a) What do you see in the first picture?
b) What has happened during orthodontic treatment?
c) How soon should traumatically intruded teeth be extruded?

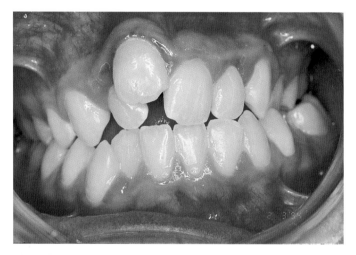

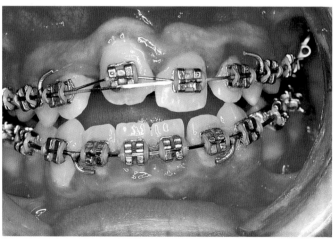

# Question 9.3

a)  What can you see here?
b)  What possible aetiological factors would you consider?
c)  How would you manage this problem?

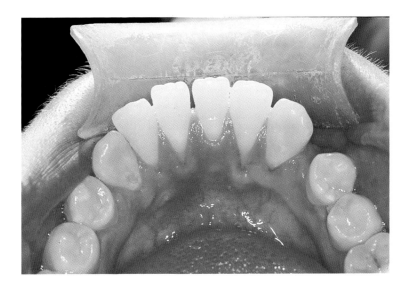

# Question 9.4

a) What has happened during orthodontic treatment?
b) Is this a common problem?
c) What are the risk factors associated with this problem?
d) How can this problem be minimized?

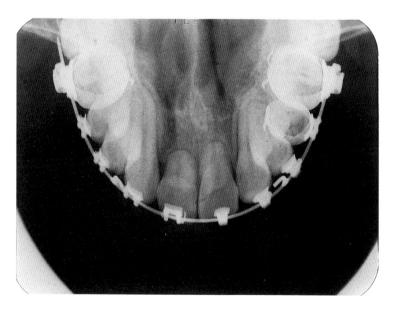

# Question 9.5

a) What do you see here and what is the cause?
b) How would you manage this problem?

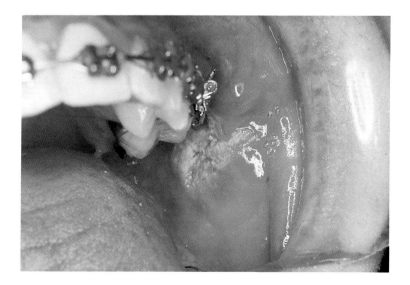

# Question 9.6

a)  What do you see here and what is the cause?
b)  How would you manage this problem?

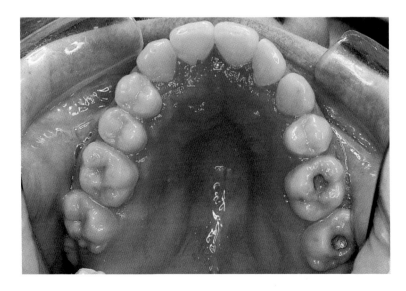

# Question 9.7

a)  What do you see here and what is the cause?
b)  How would you manage this problem?

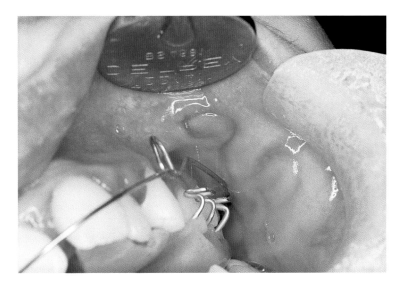

# Question 9.8

a) What do you see here and what is the cause?
b) How would you manage this problem?

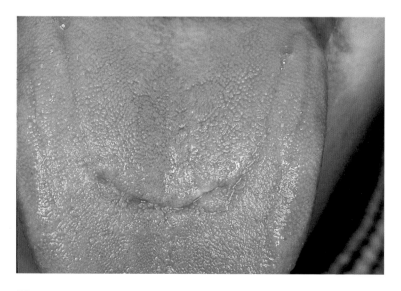

# Question 9.9

a) What do you see here?
b) What was the aim of treatment?
c) How would you manage this problem?

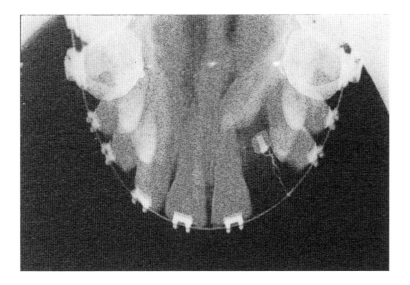

## Question 10.1

a) What appliances are these?
b) What are they for and what regime for use would you prescribe?
c) Is relapse common after orthodontic treatment? Outline some of the causes.
d) What features of the dentition pretreatment are most prone to relapse, and how can this relapse be minimized?

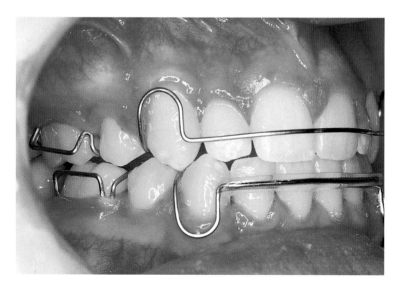

# Question 10.2

a) What appliance is attached to the lingual surfaces of the teeth?
b) What is it for and what situations might indicate its use?
c) What problems could be encountered?
d) What is the clinical procedure for making it?
e) What alternative appliances exist?
f) What is unusual about this patient's dentition?

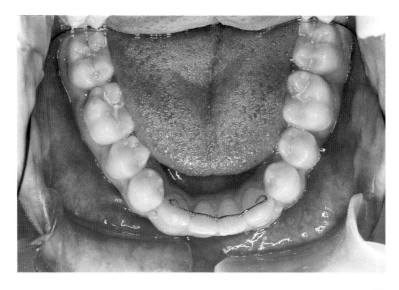

# Answers

## Answer 1.1

a)  Incisor relationship is classified as class I, II or III, depending where the lower incisors occlude relative to the cingulum plateau of the upper central incisors. This is a class I incisor relationship, where the lower incisors occlude with or lie directly below the cingulum plateau of the upper central incisors. The overjet usually measures 2–4 mm.

b)  The cusp of the upper canine occludes in the embrasure between the lower canine and first premolar, and this is called a class I canine relationship. The mesiobuccal cusp of the upper first molar occludes with the mesiobuccal groove of the lower first molar, which is an Angle's class I molar relationship. There are no crossbites or scissorbites, as the upper buccal segment teeth occlude just buccally to the opposing mandibular buccal teeth.

c)  Andrew's six keys to occlusion are based on his assessment of the study casts of 120 non-orthodontically created class I occlusions. He concluded that the six dental features common to all were:

i)  correct molar relationship
ii)  correct crown angulation
iii)  correct crown inclination
iv)  tight interproximal contacts
v)  absence of rotations
vi)  a flat curve of Spee.

Additionally, tooth size must be correctly proportioned to achieve a perfect class I occlusion. Most of these features are visible in this photograph.

d)  An Angle's class I molar relationship is such that the mesiobuccal cusp of the upper first molar occludes in the mesiobuccal groove of the lower first molar. To satisfy an Andrew's class I molar relationship, the distal cusp of the upper first molar occludes with the mesial marginal ridge of the lower second molar, i.e. supra class I Angle relationship.

# Answer 1.2

a) This photograph demonstrates canine guidance during lateral mandibular excursion.

b) This functional occlusal relationship is called mutually protected occlusion (MPO) or canine guided occlusion.

c) The mutually protected occlusion is so called because the posterior teeth protect the anterior teeth in centric occlusion, while during dynamic movements the anterior teeth protect the posterior teeth. Therefore there is minimal load placed on the anterior teeth at maximum intercuspation. Incisal guidance is seen on protrusion and canine guidance is achieved on lateral excursion. There is an immediate and gentle disclusion of the posterior teeth without occlusal interference during such movements.

d) The other main type of dynamic occlusion is called group function. In this scheme all the buccal segment teeth on the working side, rather than just the canine teeth, guide the lateral excursive movements. The non-working side teeth should not contact and, therefore, are said to be free of interference.

## Answer 2.1

a) An extraoral orthodontic examination should include:
   i) the skeletal relationship in all three planes of space
   ii) the soft tissue relationship and behaviour, especially the upper incisor/lower lip relationship
   iii) the upper incisor/upper lip relationship, both dynamically and at rest, to assess vertical maxillary excess ('gummy smile')
   iv) the dental centrelines with respect to the facial midline.
b) An intraoral orthodontic examination should include:
   i) tooth presence and quality
   ii) oral hygiene and gingival condition
   iii) lower labial segment crowding/spacing and tooth inclination
   iv) upper labial segment crowding/spacing and tooth inclination
   v) buccal segment crowding/spacing and tooth angulation
   vi) anterior occlusion i.e. overbite, overjet and upper and lower centreline coincidence
   vii) posterior occlusion i.e. canine and molar relationship, interdigitation and transverse relationships
   viii) dynamic occlusion.
c) Adjunctive procedures which may aid diagnosis include:
   i) Radiographs
   Usually a dental panoramic tomogram (DPT) to assess dental development and to detect gross pathology, and an upper occlusal view to aid localization of impacted teeth and to assess incisor root anatomy are required. A lateral cephalometric radiograph to assess skeletal relationship and tooth inclination is required for patients with a skeletal discrepancy
   ii) Study models
   iii) Photographs.

Extraoral and intraoral photographs are desirable to record facial appearance, the standard of oral hygiene and any enamel defects before treatment.

# Answer 2.2

a) This patient has a class I skeletal relationship.
b) The maxilla is positioned slightly ahead of the mandible in a class I skeletal relationship.
c) A class I skeletal relationship has an ANB value of 2–4°.
d) The skeletal vertical dimension is assessed with the patient in profile. It consists of both linear and angular measurements. Classically, the face is considered as having three equally sized proportions, although this is not precise. These facial thirds are called the upper facial third (from the top of the forehead to the soft tissue nasion); the midfacial third (from the soft tissue nasion to the base of the nose, a point called subnasale); and the lower facial third (from the subnasale to the base of the chin, a point called the menton). The midfacial and the lower facial thirds are commonly considered together, when they are referred to as the upper anterior and the lower anterior face height respectively. Collectively the two form the total anterior face height. A person with a normal facial vertical dimension has a lower anterior face height that is 55% of the total anterior face height. The Frankfort plane connects the infra-orbital rim (orbitale) to the most superior point on the external auditory meatus (porion). The lower border of the mandible forms the mandibular plane. The intersection of these two planes forms the Frankfort-mandibular planes angle that typically has a value of 27° ± 5°.

# Answer 2.3

a) This is a class I occlusion, as the canine and buccal segment teeth are class I. However, the incisors are mildly crowded and the overjet and overbite are reduced, which suggests that the incisor relationship is slightly class III. A class III incisor relationship is one where the lower incisors occlude anterior to the cingulum plateau of the upper central incisors.
b) Space to relieve crowding can be created in four ways:
   i) by extractions, the most common method of creating space

ii)   by distalization of the upper buccal segment teeth

iii)  by interdental enamel reduction, which is of use only for mildly crowded cases

iv)   by maxillary expansion, which can be considered for cases with a unilateral crossbite and a mandibular displacement on closure into centric occlusion.

All skeletal, soft tissue and dental features of the presenting malocclusion must be taken into consideration when deciding which method to use.

c)   The lower canine is distally angulated and its root needs to be moved distally using a fixed appliance. If the first premolars were extracted it is likely that the canine crown would tip even further distally if left untreated, thereby worsening the initial tooth position. This patient's treatment included the removal of all second premolars, and the provision of upper and lower fixed appliances.

# Answer 2.4

a)   This patient is in the late mixed dentition and has a class II division 1 incisor relationship. This is determined by the lower incisors which occlude palatally to the cingulum plateau of the upper incisors, while the upper incisors are proclined or of average inclination with an increased overjet. She has a mild class II skeletal relationship with a reduced vertical dimension.

b)   This type of malocclusion may be due to skeletal factors, such as mandibular retrognathia or maxillary prognathism; soft tissue factors, such as lower lip trapping or lip incompetence (lips not held together at rest); or habits, such as persistent thumb sucking.

c)   This patient presents with well-aligned, spaced arches and should be treated on a non-extraction basis. The case is very suitable for functional appliance therapy, since the patient still has growth potential and is in the mixed dentition. Therefore overjet reduction can be initiated while the permanent dentition is still being established. Additionally, this girl's teeth are not crowded and may not need fixed appliance therapy after initial treatment has successfully reduced the overjet and overbite. Fixed appliances, or an upper removable appliance, with headgear could also be successful. Whichever method is chosen, it is clear that all orthodontic treatment relies on patient co-operation for success.

# Answer 2.5

a) This patient has a mild class II skeletal relationship with increased Frankfort-mandibular planes angle and an increased lower anterior facial height. She has a pleasant soft tissue profile but incompetent lips.

b) The buccal segment relationship is ¾ unit class II, the overjet is increased and she has an anterior open bite. When the overbite is incomplete, imagine the long axis of the lower incisors and extend until it reaches the upper incisors. This shows where the lower incisors would occlude if the overbite were complete, and enables incisor classification. This is a class II division 1 incisor relationship. Buccal segment relationship is described using the Angle's classification (I, II or III). It is defined further as mild, moderate or severe by describing the cusp/embrasure discrepancy as a fraction (¼, ½, ¾, 1) of a premolar width.

c) This patient's main problem is the vertical dimension. The lower anterior facial height is increased, associated with an anterior open bite. The lip incompetence may result in a tongue to lower lip adaptive swallowing pattern, which may aggravate the anterior open bite. It is extremely important to establish control of the vertical dimension early during treatment and to ensure that the molars are not extruded. If this occurs it will make the anterior open bite and class II skeletal relationship worse. Therefore, treatment mechanics are likely to include high pull headgear to intrude the upper molars. Class II traction should be avoided, as this will extrude the lower molars.

d) The presenting malocclusion has features indicative of problems with long-term stability after treatment. The anterior open bite may relapse, as orthodontics will have only a minimal effect on the aetiological factor, the increased vertical dimension. It has been found that the greater the skeletal contribution to the open bite, the worse the prognosis for stability. A mild open bite at the start of treatment makes it more likely that the result will be stable. Overjet reduction is likely to be stable if the lips are competent at the end of treatment, with the lower lip covering the incisal third of the upper incisors at rest.

e) The gingivitis is due to poor plaque control aggravated by mouth breathing.

# Answer 2.6

a) Anteroposteriorly this patient has mandibular retrognathia and demonstrates a moderate class II skeletal relationship. She has a pleasant nose and her nasolabial angle is within normal limits at about 90°. This suggests that the maxilla is correctly positioned in the anteroposterior dimension. However, the mentalis muscle appears tense, suggesting that she can only achieve lip competence with effort, i.e. lip strain. The Frankfort-mandibular planes angle is increased and her lower anterior face height is also slightly increased. On smiling, she shows an excessive amount of upper gingivae, which demonstrates vertical maxillary excess. Her upper dental centreline is displaced to the right with respect to the facial midline, which may have been due to the early loss of the upper right deciduous canine without balancing extractions on the left.

b) In occlusion there is an increased overjet and overbite. The dental centrelines are not coincident. Her right buccal segment relationship is class I and the left buccal segment relationship is ¾ unit class II. This asymmetry is of dental, not skeletal origin since there is no facial asymmetry. The displacement of the upper centreline indicates that the right maxillary buccal segment teeth are positioned more posteriorly than the buccal segment on the left. Early loss of deciduous teeth may have contributed to the asymmetrical buccal segment relationship.

c) The upper lateral incisor teeth are small and this creates a tooth size discrepancy between the upper and lower teeth, making a normal occlusion difficult to achieve. Small upper lateral incisors can be managed in several ways:
   i)   restore them to a normal size with a composite restorative material
   ii)  close space but accept a mild class II buccal segment relationship at the end of treatment
   iii) accept slight spacing
   iv)  reduce the width of the lower incisors in accordance with a Bolton tooth size analysis.

d) Firstly, a problem list should be outlined. Her presenting problems are:
   i)   'gummy' smile (vertical maxillary excess)
   ii)  increased overjet and overbite due to mandibular retrognathia

iii)   dental asymmetry, with the upper centreline around to the right.

As an 18 year old female, her growth will have ceased, therefore orthodontic treatment cannot reduce her vertical maxillary excess or encourage her mandible to autorotate to mask her class II skeletal relationship. Therefore the 'gummy' smile and mandibular retrognathia cannot be addressed by orthodontic means alone. In order to correct the upper centreline and reduce the overjet, space will be needed from extractions in the upper arch. This might be detrimental to her facial profile, since the extraoral examination determines the anteroposterior position of the maxilla to be correct. Hence, orthodontic 'camouflage' of her class II skeletal relationship is not appropriate. In this case, the optimum management is with a combined orthodontic/orthognathic approach. This would involve a bimaxillary procedure to impact the maxilla, thereby reducing the vertical height and the amount of gingival show on smiling. This would also allow lip competence to be achieved more easily. Simultaneously the mandible would be advanced to produce a class I incisor relationship. An advancement genioplasty may also be needed to create a more normal profile.

# Answer 2.7

a)   This young boy is in the early mixed dentition and has a severe class II division 1 incisor relationship. He has a moderate class II skeletal relationship with an average vertical dimension.

b)   He has incompetent lips, due to a short upper lip. The lower lip is trapped behind the upper incisors. He has an acute nasolabial angle (normal range is 90°–110°) and a pleasing nose. The soft tissue chin point (soft tissue pogonion) is normally related to the forehead (soft tissue nasion). The soft tissue pogonion should lie within 4 mm of a vertical plane dropped from the soft tissue nasion.

c)   The principal cause of the increased overjet is the soft tissue behaviour. The upper incisors have been significantly proclined by the lower lip, which is positioned palatally to the upper labial segment at rest. This is called 'lip trapping'. The aims of treatment here are to reduce the overbite, overcome the lower lip trap and reduce the overjet. Increased mandibular growth relative to maxillary growth (which may need to be restrained through the use of headgear), or distal movement of the maxillary dentition, will compensate for the skeletal discrepancy. Successful reduction of the overjet will depend on alteration of the soft tissue behaviour. The lower lip must lie anterior to the upper incisors, the corrected position of which will be retained by lower lip control. This is achieved when the lips are competent (held together) at rest without conscious effort, i.e. without lip strain.

# Answer 2.8

a) Anteroposteriorly this patient has a class II skeletal relationship, with the mandible set back relative to the maxilla (soft tissue point B is posterior to soft tissue point A) and her Frankfort-mandibular planes angle is reduced.
b) The angle ANB is equal to or greater than 5° in a class II skeletal relationship.
c) The class II division 2 type malocclusion usually has a class II skeletal relationship, but can have skeletal I or III. The cranial base angle (formed by the lines joining nasion, sella and basion) is often obtuse which causes mandibular retrognathia, and the cranial base is long, resulting in maxillary prognathism. The maxilla is short, broad and forward relative to the mandible, which may result in a scissorbite. The lower face height is usually reduced, with reduced gonial angle and a reduced Frankfort-mandibular planes angle. A high resting lower lip line is common in this type of malocclusion, due to the reduced lower anterior face height. There is a marked labiomental fold and the masseter muscles may produce an increased bite force.
d) This patient has a strong chin, which masks her mandibular retrognathia.

# Answer 2.9

a) This photograph demonstrates a ¾ unit class II buccal segment and canine relationship. The upper incisors are very retroclined, with minimal overjet. The overbite is increased and complete to the labial gingivae with signs of trauma.
b) This is a class II division 2 incisor relationship. The lower incisor edges occlude palatally to the cingulum plateau of the upper incisors, and the upper incisors are retroclined with a

minimal overjet, although this may be increased. The retroclination of the upper incisors is the key to distinguishing
between a class II division 2 and class II division 1 incisor
relationship.

c) The key dental features of a class II division 2 malocclusion
are retroclined upper and (usually) lower incisors, which
result in an increased interincisal angle and deep overbite.
The overjet is usually reduced and the buccal segments are
often class II. A scissorbite is common in the first premolar
region, due to the broad maxilla. The crown-root angle of the
upper incisors may be reduced and they may have a poorly
defined cingulum.

d) The interincisal angle and lower incisor position, if retroclined, must be corrected after treatment to give the best
chance of stability. In order to reduce the overbite with
maximum stability, the lower incisor edges should lie anterior
to the upper incisor root centroid after treatment. Treatment
of the class II division 2 malocclusion is one of the few
instances where it is acceptable to procline the lower labial
segment. This is because the retroclined upper incisors have
caused the lower incisors to retrocline during growth, and
treatment mechanics aim to procline the lower incisors to a
normal inclination.

e) The high resting lower lip line is an aetiological factor in the
retroclination of the upper incisors. The upper lateral incisors
are often trapped on top of the lower lip, becoming mesially
angulated and mesiolabially rotated. They may need to be
pericised after treatment to increase stability.

# Answer 2.10

a) This patient has a mild class III skeletal relationship with an
increased Frankfort-mandibular planes angle, obtuse gonial
angle and increased lower anterior face height. He has an
obtuse nasolabial angle, which suggests that his maxilla is
slightly retrognathic. However, the skeletal relationship
assessment should be made in conjunction with an assessment
of the incisor inclination. If the lower incisors are found to be
retroclined, or the upper incisors proclined, then the skeletal
relationship will be more class III than appears clinically.

b) This boy has a mild class III incisor relationship with mild
crowding. The buccal segment to canine relationship is a ½
unit class III. The overjet and overbite are reduced, with the

upper right lateral incisor in crossbite with the lower right canine. The lower incisors appear to be retroclined, compensating for an underlying class III skeletal relationship.

c) The aims of orthodontic treatment of this class III malocclusion are to:
   i)   relieve the crowding
   ii)  align the teeth
   iii) correct the buccal segment relationship to class I
   iv)  if possible to increase the overjet and overbite.

   The upper incisors will need to be proclined and the lower incisors retroclined beyond average cephalometric values.

d) Unfavourable mandibular growth, especially vertically, will limit the correction of the overjet and overbite.

# Answer 2.11

a) These photographs demonstrate forwards displacement of the mandible on closure, to achieve a comfortable occlusion. The patient can reach edge to edge incisor contact, but then displaces forwards into centric occlusion. It is important to diagnose displacements on closure as this can disguise the true skeletal relationship. For example, this patient assessed in the displaced position will appear to have a more severe class III skeletal relationship than is correct. The true skeletal relationship will appear more amenable to correction orthodontically than the displaced position. A lateral mandibular displacement will suggest a facial asymmetry that is absent when the patient is assessed in the undisplaced position.

b) Patients with a class III incisor relationship usually have a class III skeletal relationship. The cranial base angle may be acute, leading to a forward position of the mandible; or the cranial base may be short, leading to maxillary retrognathia. The mandible may be large, the maxilla small or a combination of both. The maxilla tends to be small and narrow relative to the mandible, which tends to be broad. Hence crossbites are common. The gonial angle is often obtuse and the Frankfort-mandibular planes angle and lower anterior facial height are commonly increased. The pattern of mandibular growth is usually in a backward and downward direction.

c) This patient has missing upper lateral incisors, therefore the upper buccal segments are one unit forwards relative to the mandibular teeth. If the lateral incisors were present and aligned, the buccal segment relationship would be considerably more class III. Both the upper and lower incisors appear to be retroclined. The lower incisors are compensating for the underlying class III skeletal relationship, while the upper incisors have been trapped in crossbite by the lower incisors and therefore are not at their normal inclination.

## Answer 2.12

a) This patient has a class III skeletal relationship anteroposteriorly and a greatly increased lower anterior facial height. As a result, her mandibular plane is steep and the Frankfort-mandibular planes angle is increased. This is an abnormal vertical skeletal relationship.

b) The class III skeletal relationship has an ANB angle that is equal to or less than 1°.

c) In this type of skeletal relationship, the maxilla is positioned posteriorly relative to the mandible. This may be due to a small maxilla (maxillary retrognathia), or a large mandible (mandibular prognathism) or a combination of both. Alternatively, the mandible may be positioned anteriorly due to an acute cranial base angle.

d) This patient has had excessive anterior facial growth relative to the posterior facial growth. As a result, the mandible has rotated backwards (posterior growth rotation) carrying the mandibular incisors vertically away from the upper incisors. Growth of the alveolar processes has been unable to keep pace with mandibular growth and the teeth in the labial segments have achieved their full eruptive potential. This is not sufficient to achieve an overbite. The combination of these factors has resulted in the gap between the incisors. This is called an anterior open bite. Other causes of anterior open bites include habits such as thumbsucking, or soft tissue factors such as tongue size or position. However, neither of these factors was involved in the aetiology of the anterior open bite in this patient.

e) Given that the main aetiological factor in this anterior open bite is the skeletal relationship, a combination of orthodontics and orthognathic surgery is required for correction of the malocclusion.

## Answer 2.13

a) This patient has a class III skeletal relationship with increased lower anterior facial height and an increased Frankfort-mandibular planes angle.

b) In this case the buccal segment relationship demonstrates a severe class III relationship, which is greater than one full unit class III. The upper first molar only just occludes with the distal cusp of the lower first molar. The upper premolars are in crossbite with the lower first molar. In this example the lower incisors occlude anterior to the cingulum of the upper incisors. Therefore the incisor relationship is class III, demonstrating a reverse overjet and reduced overbite. The lower incisors appear to be retroclined and both upper and lower incisors are slightly imbricated.

c) The incisor relationship demonstrates the phenomenon of dentoalveolar compensation for a severe class III skeletal relationship. In an attempt to achieve a normal incisal relationship, the upper incisors have proclined. In this case the upper incisors (ui) were at 120° to the maxillary plane. The lower incisors (li) were retroclined to the mandibular plane at 72°. The compensated incisor positions have resulted in a more normal soft tissue profile than if the incisors were positioned at an average inclination to the dental bases (normal Caucasian ui/MPA = 109° ± 6°; normal Caucasian li/MnPA = 93° ± 6°). If the incisors were normally inclined, the resulting profile would show greater mandibular prognathism. This example demonstrates how tooth position can camouflage the severity of the underlying skeletal relationship.

# Answer 2.14

a) This patient has a marked mandibular asymmetry with the chin point off to the left.

b) Facial asymmetries can often worsen with continuing growth, and what might have been a mild problem at a young age can cause significant distress when the patient is older. Orthognathic surgery may be the only answer to correct the aesthetics, and it may be best to delay orthodontic treatment until it is clear that growth has slowed and the asymmetry is not worsening.

c) Mandibular displacements on closure can worsen the apparent skeletal discrepancy. As lateral displacements can give the false impression that a transverse asymmetry exists, these must be identified in order to diagnose the malocclusion correctly.

d) A lateral mandibular displacement in a child in the mixed dentition is often due to a transverse discrepancy between the maxillary and the mandibular dentition. This may be the result of a digit habit, causing upper arch narrowing and leading to a premature contact on closure. Palatal lateral incisors and deciduous canines are also common causes of occlusal interferences and thus premature contacts. Treatment often involves a combination of upper arch expansion with a removable appliance and elimination of the premature contact, or extraction of the deciduous tooth. Digit habits should be discouraged.

# Answer 2.15

a) These cases both demonstrate bimaxillary proclination where the upper and lower labial segment teeth are proclined. The incisor relationship is class I.

b) This problem is more common in afrocaribbean and oriental ethnic groups.

c) Tooth position is largely determined by the forces of the orofacial musculature at rest, i.e. the resting position of the lips and tongue. Lips that are full and everted tend to exert less pressure on the teeth than lips that are thin and strap like, pressure from the tongue is not resisted by lip pressure, and the teeth are proclined.

d) Patients with bimaxillary proclination who ask for treatment often dislike any associated spacing and sometimes complain that their 'teeth stick out'. Occasionally the overjet is increased but often it is normal and, in these cases, the patient needs to be reassured that the inclination of the teeth is not an increased overjet. Some patients also dislike their full profile and others wish to achieve lip competence.

e) The stability of treated bimaxillary proclination is variable, as retroclination of the labial segments will infringe on the tongue space. Treatment should be undertaken with caution and the patient warned in advance that long-term stability might only be possible with long-term retention. Patients who do best are those presenting with crowding and a need for premolar extractions. This relieves crowding and enables retroclination of the incisors. Premolar extractions should be avoided in spaced or aligned cases, as extraction spaces will often re-open after treatment under the influence of the tongue. Patients who are able to achieve lip competence after orthodontic treatment also have a greater chance of stability than those who had competent lips at the start of treatment. Often prolonged, indefinite retention is required.

# Answer 2.16

a)  i)  10 years
    ii)  11.5 ± 2 years.
b)  The deciduous canines are retained in the arch and all other permanent teeth, except third molars, have erupted. In this case the permanent canines were impacted palatally.
c)  Palpate the canine region to assess the canine position. If it cannot be determined, take parallax radiographs (DPT and upper occlusal view, or two periapical films from different angles) to do so. If it alters in the same direction as the Xray tube shift, then it lies palatally. If the canine moves in the opposite direction to the tube shift, then it lies buccally. If there is no change, then it is in the line of the arch. This method of identifying tooth position can be remembered as the 'SLOB' (same lingual, opposite buccal) rule.
d)  There are many factors to take into account when treatment planning for this problem. These include:
    i)   patient age and attitude towards treatment
    ii)  state of general and dental health
    iii) presenting malocclusion
    iv)  position of the canine and the severity of the impaction
    v)   root resorption of teeth adjacent to the canine
    vi)  extent of crowding
    vii) lateral incisor/premolar contact.
    In general terms, the greater the malposition of the canine (e.g. lying horizontally, with the crown near the midline), the lesser the chance of successful alignment orthodontically. The position of the canine root apex must be favourable.

    If the canines are normally positioned then no treatment is necessary, although extraction of the deciduous canines should be considered to hasten eruption of the permanent canines. If the canines are impacted, the following should be considered:

## Interceptive management

For a child aged 10–13 years with uncrowded arches, extract the deciduous canines and maintain or create space for normalization of the upper canines. This is successful in 78% of cases presenting with palatally impacted upper permanent canines.

### Active management to align the canines

The impacted canines can be exposed surgically and aligned using an orthodontic appliance. Some clinicians prefer a gold chain to be bonded to the canines at the time of surgery and the mucosal flap to be replaced. If the canines are buccally positioned and high, then apically repositioned flaps for exposure are not feasible. These malpositioned canines require a flap to be raised and then a bond with a gold chain to be attached to the canine. A fixed appliance is used to apply traction to the chain, which brings the tooth down into position.

### Surgical removal of the impacted canines

Removal is a realistic option if the canines are very unfavourably positioned and lateral incisor/premolar contact exists or can be created orthodontically.

### Passive management

Impacted canines can be kept under radiographic observation. This is not the ideal solution as the deciduous canines will eventually be lost and prosthetic replacement will need to be considered.

# Answer 2.17

a) This is a postoperative photograph of palatally impacted permanent canines that have been surgically exposed. This allows access to bond an attachment, such as a bracket or eyelet, which can then be used to apply traction to the impacted teeth. Additionally, this patient has molar separators in place prior to placing molar bands. An alternative method of managing impacted canines is by direct bonding with eyelet and gold chain and flap replacement at the time of surgery. In contrast, surgically exposing the crown rather than the gold chain approach has two important advantages. Firstly, as the tooth is bonded postoperatively a dry field should be easier to achieve and so the bond may be more successful. Secondly, if the bond fails it is rapidly noticed and repaired. However, in the hands of an inexperienced surgeon, incomplete exposure may be made and the canines may quickly be covered by granulation tissue.

b) Impacted maxillary canines occur in approximately 2% of the population.

c) This problem is more common in females, with a ratio of females:males of 85:15.

d) Several factors are associated with impacted maxillary canines: it is a familial condition, predominating in females, and there are associations with class II division 2 malocclusions and small or missing upper lateral incisors.

e) Root resorption of the upper lateral incisors will occur in 12% of cases with impacted maxillary canines, especially in girls under 14 years of age. In severe cases, the roots of the upper central incisors can also be resorbed.

# Answer 2.18

a) This is a lateral open bite, also known as posterior open bite.

b) This rare condition has a number of possible causes, which may be of skeletal, soft tissue or dental origin. It may be a combination of all three. Often the skeletal vertical dimension will be increased and development of the alveolar process will not have kept pace. Rarely, unilateral condylar hyperplasia may be the cause. The tongue (as in this case) may spread laterally, preventing full tooth eruption. This may be due to the tongue being large or to premature loss of the first molars allowing the tongue to spread into the extraction space. Finally, it may arise from an inherent failure of tooth eruption. This may be due to primary failure of eruption or arrested tooth eruption.

c) It is important to be sure that the affected teeth are not ankylosed, as these cannot be extruded orthodontically. The net effect could be intrusion of the adjacent, unaffected teeth. Ankylosed teeth have a distinctive sound when percussed, that is duller than adjacent teeth. It is important to check this before starting and during treatment. Additionally, careful measurement of the lateral open bite should be made at each visit as a progress check, and adjacent tooth position should be monitored to ensure that the overbite is maintained.

# Answer 2.19

a)  This is a child in the early mixed dentition who has an asymmetrical anterior open bite and unilateral crossbite tendency. The fraenal attachment is low and fibrous and may be contributing to the diastema.

b)  The asymmetrical nature of the malocclusion suggests that the aetiology is a persistent habit, in this instance thumb sucking.

c)  Digit sucking has several effects on the dentition and the skeletal relationship. Generally the overjet is increased and asymmetrical, while the overbite is reduced and incomplete. The tongue is displaced by the thumb and so held at a lower position than normal. Without tongue pressure, the maxilla narrows and a unilateral crossbite tendency is common. A lateral mandibular displacement on closure may be present. The mandible is held open, resulting in excessive eruption of the posterior teeth, a backward growth rotation and a more class II skeletal relationship.

d)  This child initially needs to be encouraged to stop thumb sucking. Sometimes an explanation may be sufficient. When the permanent dentition is more established an upper removable appliance can be fitted to expand the upper arch, and this may stop the habit. Fixed habit breakers, such as the hayrake appliance, may be considered. Committed thumb suckers will carry on regardless. Finally, white cotton gloves, available from chemists, will help to stop a night-time habit.

# Answer 2.20

a)  This is a child in the early mixed dentition with the upper central incisors trapped in crossbite with the lower central incisors, which are labially displaced and demonstrate gingival recession. This is called an anterior crossbite.

b)  This is a significant problem, as the periodontal attachment of the lower incisors can be damaged.

c)  The upper incisors need to be proclined with an upper removable appliance. The lower incisors may need to be actively retroclined.

d)  Various designs are possible for this problem.
    This is the design used in an upper removable appliance:
    i)   cantilever springs behind the upper incisors in 0.7 mm stainless steel wire

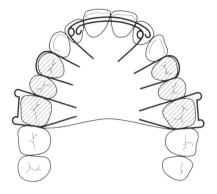

ii)     Adams cribs on the upper first permanent molars in
        0.7 mm stainless steel wire and Jackson's cribs on the
        deciduous first molars in 0.6 mm stainless steel wire
iii)    posterior bite capping
iv)     baseplate.

## Answer 2.21

a) The right maxillary canine and first premolar have been transposed.
b) Transpositions are not a common problem, but they almost
   always involve the canine. Transposition of the canine and
   first premolar is the most frequently occurring (71% of
   recorded cases). It is more common in females than males and
   is more frequent on the left.
c) The root position of the affected teeth has a major influence
   upon the decision whether or not to accept the transposition.
   Sometimes only the crowns have changed position and this is
   described as a pseudotransposition, which is easier to correct.
   If the roots have transposed, then their position is best
   accepted. Other factors that influence treatment planning are
   the degree of crowding, type of malocclusion and patient
   motivation.
d) The aetiological factors contributing to this problem include
   the early loss of deciduous teeth and genetic predisposition.

# Answer 2.22

a) The upper right central incisor is missing and space has been lost. Investigations should determine if it is impacted or has been avulsed, as in this case.

b) Space maintenance before orthodontic treatment can be difficult, especially if the incisor is lost at a young age. An upper removable appliance (URA) with an artificial tooth should be provided. It is optimistic to expect acrylic alone to preserve the space entirely. Although wires detract from aesthetics, C clasps mesial and distal to the missing tooth will give the best chance of total space maintenance.

c) The best aesthetic effect during orthodontic treatment is achieved by maintaining the URA as a spoon denture for as long as possible. Alternatively, an acrylic tooth may be bonded with a bracket and ligated to the archwire. This is difficult with the initial light wires since the acrylic tooth tends to spin on the wire. If the incisor is lost during active treatment, then it can be decoronated and a bracket bonded to the enamel. The natural crown may then be ligated to the wire.

d) Definitive restorative options should be discussed with the dentist, who will provide the restorative treatment before orthodontic treatment begins. The dilemma at the start of treatment is whether to open or close the space. It is possible to bring the lateral incisor into the central incisor position and then crown it to mimic the central incisor. The aesthetics of this are rarely satisfactory as the gingival margin and crown contour look abnormal, although adhesive composite restoration can mask this to a degree. The best aesthetic result will be achieved by opening the space and providing an artificial replacement. Options include:

## Denture

This is satisfactory in the short term while the dentition becomes fully established, but for a single tooth replacement it is not ideal.

## Bridgework

Conventional bridgework involves crowning adjacent teeth to support the pontic. This is very destructive and is only indicated if the adjacent teeth are heavily restored. Adhesive bridgework is preferred, providing the overbite allows for the placement of metal wings. In general, a cantilever design has the greatest success rate.

## Implant

Single tooth implants are increasingly more popular. However, they are expensive and cannot be used until growth has ceased, since implants do not erupt with continued alveolar development.

The final restoration must be considered carefully at the start of treatment, since space requirements are different for each option. For example, the pontic space required for an adhesive bridge is less than that needed for an implant.

# Answer 2.23

a) This patient, in the early mixed dentition, has infraoccluded deciduous molars and an anterior open bite. The first molars are the only teeth in occlusion.
b) The deciduous molars have become ankylosed. Teeth become ankylosed when the process of resorption and repair becomes imbalanced. As deciduous teeth are shed, their roots undergo resorption and repair simultaneously. If the rate of repair exceeds resorption then the roots can fuse to surrounding bone. As the surrounding teeth and alveolar processes continue to develop normally, the ankylosed teeth are left behind and become infraoccluded. Commonly single teeth (usually second deciduous molars) are affected and this is often due to the lack of a permanent successor. However, in this case, where several teeth in each arch are affected, there appears to be a generalised disturbance in eruption and the affected teeth may never have reached the level of the normal occlusal plane. This is referred to as a primary failure of eruption.
c) If the deciduous molars have an eruption disturbance then the prognosis for the permanent dentition is poor, as it is likely that it will be similarly affected. It is not possible to extrude affected teeth orthodontically. Therefore a restorative approach to build up the teeth to the level of the occlusal plane or to provide an overdenture may need to be considered.
d) The anterior open bite may be due to:
   i) skeletal factors e.g. increased lower anterior face height
   ii) soft tissue factors e.g. forwards tongue posture or atypical swallowing pattern

iii)    habits e.g. digit sucking
iv)    a combination of the above.

# Answer 2.24

a)  The upper right central incisor is missing and space loss has occurred. There is contact between the upper left central and upper right lateral incisors. The upper left central incisor has drifted to the right across the dental midline and has displaced the labial fraenum.
b)  This problem should be investigated by:

## Taking a full history

Has the tooth previously been extracted or avulsed? Is there a history of trauma to the deciduous predecessor?

## Dental and orthodontic examination

Is the missing incisor palpable? What is the standard of dental health? What are the other presenting features of the malocclusion?

## Radiographs

Radiographs identify the presence and position of the impacted tooth and also identify any associated pathology. In order to use the parallax method of identification to identify the position of the missing tooth, radiographs should be taken in two planes. A dental panoramic tomogram and standard upper occlusal view would be ideal. Alternatively, if clinical interest is focused only on the upper incisor region, then two periapical radiographs, taken at different angles, would suffice.

c)  Firstly a diagnosis must be established, as the upper right central incisor could be missing or impacted. If it has been lost, then a decision needs to be made as to whether to keep the existing malocclusion and disguise it by restorative means, or to open space for replacement of the central incisor. Full discussion with a restorative dentist, the patient and parents must be undertaken before a decision is reached. In fact, in this instance the tooth was impacted. The management of this problem is dependent on many variables, which need to be considered collectively. These include patient motivation, degree of tooth impaction, presenting dental health and malocclusion, quality of the impacted and adjacent teeth (e.g. is the root dilacerated or resorbed?) and the standard of available surgical and restorative support. In general, the treatment options to be considered for the impacted tooth are as follows.

## Alignment

Expose surgically and bond the impacted incisor, or use a gold chain and replacement flap procedure, before aligning the impacted tooth with fixed appliances.

## Removal

The impacted tooth could be removed and the lateral incisor built up to mimic the central incisor. This is not the best aesthetic option, but it does avoid the need for orthodontic treatment. Alternatively space could be created orthodontically for the restorative replacement of the central incisor.

## Transplantation

This is dependent upon the impacted tooth being removed intact.

## No active intervention

Keep the impacted tooth under periodic radiographic review. Space to accommodate the impacted incisor will need to be created orthodontically beforehand if it is to be aligned or transplanted.

d) Aetiological factors which may have caused this problem include:
   i) Trauma e.g. in the deciduous dentition trauma can result in damage to the permanent tooth germ, which may develop a dilacerated root and fail to erupt
   ii) Midline supernumerary
   iii) Pathology e.g. dentigerous cyst.

# Answer 2.25

a) This radiograph demonstrates hypodontia.

b) This patient is missing upper lateral incisors, lower central incisors, the lower left lateral incisor, lower second premolars and all third molars.

c) The most commonly missing teeth in the Caucasian population are third molars (25%), second premolars (3%) and upper lateral incisors (2%).

d) Lower central incisors are the most commonly missing teeth in the Japanese population.

e) Cleft lip and palate, Down's syndrome, hypohidrotic ectodermal dysplasia and orofacial digital syndrome are all associated with missing teeth. However, most patients with hypodontia do not have additional abnormalities.

# Answer 2.26

a) This photograph demonstrates missing upper lateral incisors. The maxillary canines are in contact with the upper central incisors.

b) The incidence of developmentally missing upper lateral incisors is about 2%.

c) The main decision to be made is whether to open space and provide prosthetic replacements for the lateral incisors, or to keep the canines alongside the central incisors as shown here. This decision can only be made after a number of factors have been taken into consideration. These include:
   i) the presenting malocclusion
   ii) colour and shape of the canines
   iii) the available restorative back-up and who will bear the long-term cost
   iv) patient motivation.

d) The maxillary canines can be aesthetically modified by:
   i) grinding, e.g. the cusp tip can be ground to create an incisal edge
   ii) restorative build-up, e.g. composite added to the labial aspect or incisal edges of the canines can improve their appearance
   iii) position, e.g. the tip and torque expressed by a pre-angulated pre-torqued bracket can be manipulated by altering bracket position to move the canine, so that it resembles a lateral incisor.

# Answer 2.27

a) This overbite is increased and complete to the palate. The inflamed palatal mucosa has been stripped from the left upper central and lateral incisors, resulting in exposure of the root. This is called a traumatic overbite. Additionally, the upper left central incisor is discoloured and has a palatal restoration, suggesting that it has been root-treated.

b) The deep overbite is caused by skeletal disproportion, commonly mandibular retrognathia, with the lower incisors set back further than is ideal. As a result they occlude with the hard palate or the gingival margin instead of the cingulum plateau of the upper incisors. The accumulation of plaque causes a deep overbite to become traumatic.

c) A regime of meticulous oral hygiene should be established and the problem kept under review. Reduction of the overbite should be considered and in a growing child is usually straightforward, but in an adult may be achievable only through orthognathic surgery.

## Answer 3.1

a) General aims of orthodontic treatment are to:
   i)   relieve crowding
   ii)  level, align and co-ordinate the dental arches
   iii) correct the canine relationship to class I
   iv)  correct the overbite and overjet
   v)   correct the buccal segment relationship to maximum intercuspation
   vi)  close space
   vii) retain.

b) In general, orthodontic treatment aims to establish a class I incisal relationship. With the teeth at normal inclination, this can be achieved only if the underlying skeletal relationship is, or is very nearly, class I in the anteroposterior plane. If the skeletal relationship is not class I, then it needs to be corrected, or the tooth inclination needs to be manipulated to disguise the underlying skeletal discrepancy. This is called orthodontic camouflage and is at its most successful if the skeletal discrepancy is mild. Therefore, when a patient is assessed, the clinician must decide if the existing skeletal relationship will allow a normal incisor relationship to be achieved or if the skeletal relationship must be modified. This can be attempted through choice of treatment mechanics, such as the application of headgear, or through orthognathic surgery at the end of growth. It must be stressed that the alteration of the skeletal relationship through non-surgical means is achievable only to a limited extent. Often correction of a class II skeletal relationship has occurred simply because a patient has grown favourably and not because the ortho-dontist has been able to influence growth.

   Vertically, the skeletal relationship influences the degree of overbite found. Therefore a patient with a reduced vertical dimension tends to have an increased overbite, and treatment planning must include how this overbite will be reduced. Conversely, a patient with an increased vertical dimension and reduced overbite will need to be treatment planned carefully so that the overbite is not further reduced by the treatment mechanics.

Finally, to achieve good facial aesthetics and maximal buccal segment interdigitation, the upper and lower dental centrelines must be coincident with each other and the facial midline. Therefore, the transverse skeletal plane must be assessed for underlying asymmetry and also for cants in the occlusal planes which would indicate asymmetrical growth. If asymmetry exists, treatment is best delayed until growth has ceased and then a decision can be made as to whether it is to be accepted, with compromised facial and occlusal appearance, or treated by surgical means.

c) Multiple factors influence the decision as to whether or not dental extractions are required to treat a malocclusion. However, patients with a reduced vertical dimension will have more difficulties with mandibular space closure than those with an increased vertical dimension. Therefore, in general, mandibular extractions should be avoided where possible for patients with a reduced vertical dimension.

# Answer 3.2

a) Growth potential is significant when assessing unfavourable features of the presenting skeletal relationship. For example, mandibular growth will help the correction of a class II skeletal relationship, but will hinder camouflage of a class III skeletal relationship. Growth will help reduce a deep overbite but may worsen a reduced overbite. Likewise, an asymmetry is likely to worsen if further growth is to occur. Therefore, potential growth must be considered when planning treatment. For example, treatment of a class II malocclusion will be aided by growth, while treatment of a high angle class III case and those cases with asymmetry is best delayed until growth has slowed and the clinician can truly assess the final malocclusion.

b) Treatment aims that are most helped by favourable growth are the reduction of overbite and overjet, and space closure.

c) There is considerable individual variation in the timing of the pubertal growth spurt. It is nearly two years earlier in girls than in boys. Girls tend to have a growth spurt at 10.5–12.5 years and boys at 12.5–14.5 years.

d) Growth studies have established that both jaws rotate during growth. A backward mandibular growth rotation is described when the mandibular border and chin point rotate downward and backward. This is important because it will:

i) worsen a class II skeletal relationship, as B point on the mandible is carried further behind A point on the maxilla

ii) reduce the overbite

iii) alter treatment mechanics, which should be aimed at minimising unwanted effects. A backward rotation is worsened by mandibular molar extrusion. Class II traction, which extrudes lower molars, should be avoided if possible and maxillary molars can be actively intruded to encourage rotation of the mandible in a forward direction.

# Answer 3.3

a) A normal overbite is important for satisfactory masticatory function, i.e. ensuring separation of the posterior teeth during mandibular protrusion and facilitating incision. Overbite is also important for stability following the correction of anterior crossbites. Ideally, the upper incisors should overlap the incisal third of the lower incisors and the lower incisal edges should occlude with the palatal cingulum of the upper incisors.

b) The vertical skeletal dimension and degree of overbite are inversely related. As the anterior face height increases, the overbite decreases. Eventually the alveolar processes reach the limits of growth and tooth eruption fails to compensate for the increased vertical dimension, and an open bite may result. Conversely, people with reduced anterior face height are likely to have a deep overbite, as the alveolar processes are closer together.

c) The overbite must be reduced before the overjet can be reduced.

d) Overbite reduction can occur in two ways, i.e. by extrusion of buccal segment teeth or intrusion of the incisors. Often it is achieved by a combination of both. Tooth extrusion does require bony support and alveolar basal bone growth occurs with greater volume and speed in a growing child than in adult patients.

e) Overbite reduction may be achieved by:

i)     the anterior bite plane of a removable appliance, which allows mandibular molar eruption

ii)    molar eruption while the incisors are held in a class I relationship with a functional appliance

iii)   correction of the interincisal angle in deep bite cases with retroclined incisors. This reduces the overbite automatically

iv)    extrusion of mandibular molars with class II traction exerted on a fixed appliance

v)     incorporating all lower molars into a fixed appliance

vi)    applying curves of Spee to upper archwires and reverse curves of Spee to lower archwires

vii)   J hook headgear to intrude the upper incisors (although this does increase root resorption) or cervical pull headgear to extrude the maxillary molars

viii)  segmental intrusion mechanics with a fixed appliance

ix)    surgical levelling.

# Answer 3.4

a)  Crowding occurs when the space required to align the teeth is greater than the space available. This is called a space discrepancy. Mild crowding exists when the space discrepancy is 4 mm or less, a moderately crowded case has a space discrepancy of 5–8 mm and a severely crowded case has a space discrepancy of 9 mm or more. Both upper canines are excluded buccally in this patient, therefore 18 mm of space is required to align them. A little space will be available once the upper second deciduous molar is lost, but this will be insufficient to accommodate the canines. This case is severely crowded and will need upper arch extractions.

b)  i)    class I
    ii)   class III
    iii)  class II.

c)  Many factors must be taken into consideration when planning dental extractions. These can be classified as extraoral and intraoral factors. Extraoral factors are:

    i)    skeletal relationship, e.g. avoid lower arch extractions in cases with reduced vertical dimension

    ii)   soft tissue profile, especially the nasolabial angle. An obtuse nasolabial angle may be worsened by retraction of the upper incisors. Therefore it may be desirable to avoid upper premolar extractions if possible in these patients

iii)  growth potential e.g. lower arch extractions should be avoided in skeletal III cases in whom growth is still active, as this may compromise future orthodontic decompensation for orthognathic surgery.

Intraoral factors are:

i)  tooth number and quality, e.g. first premolars should not be removed without ensuring that the second premolars are present and in a good position

ii)  degree and site of crowding

iii)  magnitude of overbite and overjet

iv)  dental centreline position relative to the facial midline

v)  anchorage requirements

vi)  the planned buccal segment relationship at the end of treatment. For instance, bilateral extractions in the lower arch only in a patient with a full complement of permanent teeth will create a class III buccal segment relationship, with unopposed terminal upper molars. Therefore it is usually preferable to extract in the upper arch also, to keep the buccal segment relationship class I

vii)  pathology, e.g. impacted canines may be too severely malpositioned to align orthodontically and may be extracted

viii)  incisor inclination, e.g. extractions may be required for decompensation prior to orthognathic surgery.

# Answer 3.5

a)  In general, treatment planning starts with the lower arch. In order to maximise treatment stability the inclination of the lower labial segment should be the same at the beginning and at the end of treatment. Therefore treatment planning should start with how to manage the lower arch malocclusion, while maintaining the lower incisors at their initial labiolingual inclination. Two principal exceptions to this general rule are class II division 2 cases and those with a digit habit. This is because the lower incisors have been artificially retroclined from their natural labiolingual position. Some clinicians start treatment planning by assessing the lower incisor position relative to the aesthetic line, A point to pogonion (APo), as it is thought that the best profile is achieved when the lower incisors rest on this line. However, this is not a guide to maximal stability.

b) The mandibular intercanine and intermolar widths are generally not altered during treatment since they usually relapse to their initial positions.

# Answer 3.6

a) This child is in the early mixed dentition.
b) The position of the upper permanent canines should be diagnosed by the age of 10 years. If they are not palpable in the buccal sulcus by this age then radiographic examination should be performed.
c) Early unilateral loss of a deciduous canine is likely to cause a shift of the centreline to the affected side, and this will prevent an ideal buccal segment interdigitation being achieved in the permanent dentition. An upper centreline shift can be very unaesthetic. The effects of early loss of deciduous teeth are most pronounced in crowded cases.
d) Early unilateral loss of a deciduous second molar is likely to cause the permanent dentition to appear to be crowded and the succeeding second premolar may become impacted.
e) Extraction of the deciduous canine on the affected side, and space creation if the case is crowded, will help to normalise a maxillary permanent canine that appears to be palatally positioned.

# Answer 3.7

a) Unilateral extractions can cause or worsen malocclusion due to centreline shifts and the development of asymmetrical buccal segment occlusion. A balancing extraction is made to preserve symmetry and limit adverse effects on the developing occlusion. Early unilateral loss of a deciduous canine or first deciduous molar has the greatest effect on the centreline and should be balanced by loss of a contralateral deciduous tooth.
b) A similar principle applies when teeth are lost in one arch only and an extraction is required in the opposing arch in order to limit deleterious effects on the occlusion. This is called a compensating extraction. For example, loss of a mandibular first molar prior to the eruption of the lower second molar may result in the maxillary first molar overerupting. Therefore, consideration should be given to loss of

the maxillary first molar at the same time. All the presenting features of the occlusion should be considered when planning extractions.

c)  There are no rigid guidelines to follow when considering space maintenance and it should be planned for the benefit of the individual. However, in general, space should be maintained for avulsed upper central incisors and impacted canines following the loss of the deciduous canine. When deciduous molars are lost, a decision should be based on the child's likely need for extractions of permanent teeth in the future. If the child will not need extractions, or if the teeth will be severely crowded so that every millimetre of extraction space will be needed to treat the malocclusion, then space maintenance will be helpful. However, if extractions will be needed and the case is not severely crowded, then space maintenance is not necessary. Loss of deciduous molars is usually due to caries. If this is the case, long-term space maintenance in a caries prone mouth may cause further harm.

# Answer 3.8

a)  A lateral cephalometric radiograph is a sagittal view of the patient's skeletal and facial structures taken in a standardised manner, with the patient's head placed in a cephalostat. The patient is positioned at a distance of 2 m from the Xray beam and less than 0.3 m from the film, with the Frankfort plane parallel to the floor and the head held in position by the ear rods of the cephalostat. The midsagittal plane of the patient is parallel with the plane of the film and the patient must bite together in undisplaced centric occlusion. The central Xray beam is perpendicular to the sagittal plane and is centred to the middle of the film. If these distances are varied, then the magnification of the final image is distorted. There is always some magnification, but this should be standardized between 5–12%. Some operators prefer to position the patient using natural head posture rather than the Frankfort plane, as this may allow greater reproducibility for subsequent images of the same patient.

b)  Lateral cephalometric radiographs supplement the clinical examination. They are used as a means of assessing the hard and soft tissue relationships of the patient's facial structure. The upper and lower incisor and inter-incisor angulation is also assessed. Various analyses have been created which

compare the patient's values to normal values for the appropriate population. This enables the clinician to assess the
severity of the patient's malocclusion compared with the
normal population group, and aids treatment planning. In
addition to diagnosis and treatment planning, cephalometry
may be used to predict the likely growth pattern to be experienced by the patient, and may be used as a research tool.

c) Care should be taken to minimise radiation dosage and
ensure a good quality film. As the image is taken, appropriate exposure and radiation dose settings should be used. Rare
earth screens must be employed to reduce the intensity of
radiation needed to generate an image. An aluminium wedge
between the patient and the Xray tube will enhance the soft
tissue profile by minimizing 'burn out' of the soft tissues. Xray
scatter can be reduced by placing a grid over the film cassette.
However, this tends not to be needed with modern machines.
Finally, careful developing techniques will maximise image
quality.

# Answer 3.9

a) Anteroposteriorly, the skeletal relationship is severely class
III, demonstrated by the ANB difference of $-12°$. The maxillary mandibular planes angle is $15°$, which is significantly
reduced compared to the normal of $27°$ and shows that the
patient's skeletal relationship is reduced in the vertical plane.

b) The lower incisors are upright at $80°$ to the mandibular plane.
The normal angulation is $93° \pm 6°$. The upper incisors are very
proclined at $133°$ relative to the norm of $109° \pm 6°$. These
normal values depend on which populations they are drawn
from. In this case Caucasian norms were appropriate, but the
patient's incisor angulations are extreme for any population
group. The incisors have tipped beyond normal values in an
attempt to overcome the severe class III skeletal relationship.
This is an example of dentoalveolar compensation.

c) The overjet is reversed, but the incisors are almost edge to
edge, therefore the reverse overjet is small. This is surprising
in view of the severity of the underlying skeletal relationship
and is because the incisors have attempted to compensate.

d) The value for SNA is $81.5°$ and this is essentially normal,
showing that the maxilla is correctly positioned. Therefore,
much of the skeletal III relationship can be attributed to a
large mandible.

e) The severity of the skeletal relationship and the degree of dentoalveolar compensation already present indicates that a normal overjet and overbite will not be achievable by orthodontic means alone. Therefore, a combined orthodontic and orthognathic approach will be required if the patient wishes to have treatment.

# Answer 3.10

a) The incisor relationship is a class II division 2, where the lower incisors occlude palatal to the cingulum plateau of retroclined upper incisors. The overbite is increased.
b) The maxillary position is normal with an SNA of 81.5°. This suggests that much of the malocclusion is due to a small or retropositioned mandible.
c) The upper incisors are retroclined at 99° but the lower incisors are slightly proclined at 98°. Therefore there has been some dentoalveolar compensation for a moderately severe skeletal II relationship. In a class II division 2 type malocclusion the overjet is usually within normal limits or reduced; here it is slightly increased at 6 mm (the norm for the population is 3 ± 1 mm) due to the underlying anteroposterior skeletal discrepancy. In fact, the overjet should be even greater, but has been minimised by the compensated incisor positions. This can lead to underestimation of the severity of the skeletal relationship and demonstrates that incisor angulation must be carefully considered at diagnosis.

# Answer 3.11

a) IOTN stands for the Index Of Treatment Need and PAR stands for Peer Assessment Rating.
b) The difference between these indices are that the IOTN assesses the need for treatment while the PAR Index is a means of measuring the improvement achieved by a course of orthodontic treatment.
c) The Index of Treatment Need is divided into a dental health component (DHC), which is further subdivided into five categories, and an aesthetic component (AC) which has ten categories. The DHC is the main guide to determining treatment need. A Grade 1 has no need for treatment and Grade 5 has the greatest need. Within this latter group are patients

with cleft lip and/or palate, overjets greater than 9 mm, reverse overjets greater than 3.5 mm, missing teeth with restorative implications, supernumerary teeth and impacted teeth (not third molars).

## Answer 4.1

a) This is a unilateral cleft lip and palate.

b) Clefting in humans occurs in approximately 1 in 700 live births although this varies depending on race. In black races there is a very low incidence, whereas in races from South East Asia the incidence is much higher (1 in 500 live births). The prevalence of unilateral cleft lip and palate within the cleft population varies between 16 and 25%, depending on the population examined.

c) The aetiology of clefting is not known. There is a genetic element, but this is not fully understood. There are familial tendencies but apart from one Icelandic family where clefting was X-linked, no clear association has been found. Clefts of the palate are seen in a significant number of head and neck syndromes. Anti-epileptic drugs, such as phenytoin, are associated with clefting, as is the acne drug Roaccutane (isotretinoin), which should be avoided during pregnancy. High doses of vitamin A have caused experimentally induced cleft palates in rodents.

d) The timing of palatal shelf elevation is critical. In the human embryo this occurs at 6–8 weeks. The elevation of the shelves happens remarkably quickly (usually within 24 hours) and depends on the shelves elevating above the tongue. This may require the tongue to drop. The mechanisms of shelf elevation which have been postulated are as follows.

### An increase in vascularity at the tips of the shelves

This may increase their rigidity, causing them to elevate.

## An increased accumulation of proteoglycan at the palatal shelf tips

These molecules can absorb enormous amounts of water, increasing the turgidity that again may cause the shelves to elevate.

## Contraction of collagen

An 'intrinsic' force is thought to be generated and this may cause the shelves to elevate. The mechanism is not fully understood.

After shelf elevation, formation of the palate is dependent upon removal of the medial edge epithelium (through apoptosis, programmed cell death or epithelial mesenchymal transformation), mesenchyme flow and development of myogenic and osteogenic blastemata.

# Answer 4.2

a) Expression of clefting in humans may be divided as follows.

## Clefts of the lip (unilateral or bilateral)

The clefts are described as being complete if there is no union. Expression varies from a simple notching to a complete cleft. The alveolus may or may not be affected.

## Clefts of the palate

These are divided into those of the hard or the soft palate. Clefting in the soft palate can vary from a simple bifid uvula to a complete cleft. There may also be a submucous cleft where the hard palate is cleft but the soft palate is intact. This may first be detected by speech therapists since these patients often have hypernasal speech. Clefts of the hard palate have variable expression. They are either complete or incomplete and may or may not involve the alveolus. Various classifications have been suggested. None have been universally accepted although a written classification offers a great deal.

b) The surgical management of cleft lip and palate depends on the severity of the anomaly. Management is always a compromise between function and aesthetics. Surgery restores function, enabling the child to eat without nasal regurgitation and to speak more clearly. However, the scarring affects facial growth to a variable degree. In populations where unoperated clefts have survived into adulthood, facial growth is not normally compromised. The timings of surgical repair vary between hospital specialist units. However, the general timings for closure of various aspects of the cleft are as follows.

## Lip closure at 3 months

If the condition is bilateral, some surgeons repair one side and then the other 4 weeks later. Others prefer to close the lip (and in some cases the lip and palate) at 24–48 hours after birth. There is no good evidence that this technique has any beneficial effects and the consequences of early scarring are likely to compromise normal facial growth. However, proponents of neonatal surgery suggest that it is of great psychological benefit for the parents of a cleft child.

## The hard and soft palates usually at 9 months

Hard palate closure involves mobilizing palatal mucosa across the cleft. There is no repair of the bony defect. In some units there has been a vogue for delayed closure of the hard palate until 7 or 8 years of age. This was found to result in very poor speech but good facial growth.

## Alveolar bone grafting

Grafting is carried out when the root of the permanent canine is two thirds formed (at 10–12 years of age). Autogenous bone (usually from the hip) is grafted into the alveolus. This provides bone into which the canine can erupt and it also stabilises the major and minor segments of unilateral or bilateral clefts.

## Orthognathic surgery

Patients who have not experienced favourable facial growth may need orthognathic surgery once growth has ceased. This is usually around the age of 18 years, although mid-face osteogenic dystraction may be performed at a younger age.

# Answer 4.3

a)  All types of cleft may be associated with abnormalities in the dentition. It is not uncommon to find a number of permanent teeth missing, particularly the second premolars. Paradoxically, supernumerary teeth may form in the cleft site. Presumably the disruption of the dental lamina in the cleft site creates 'satellites' which produce tooth germs. The morphology of the teeth may be altered and frequently the crowns are smaller in cleft children than in the non-cleft population.

b)  It is vital that teeth are preserved in cleft patients. Therefore a routine of regular dental care and good oral hygiene should be established from an early age. Appropriate fluoride supplementation is essential for the developing dentition and all first molars should be fissure sealed.

# Answer 4.4

a)  This is a labial fraenum, which is attached in an abnormal, low position.

b)  It can cause and maintain a diastema between the upper central incisors and prevent them being completely approximated. After orthodontic treatment, a fleshy fraenum can cause a diastema to reopen. It can also impede oral hygiene and may be considered unsightly.

c)  In order for the teeth to be properly approximated, this fraenum needs to be surgically removed. If removed prior to orthodontic treatment, full access to the surgical site is possible and the fibrous attachments to the interdental bone can be completely removed. However, it is also argued that the resultant scar tissue makes tooth movement difficult since teeth are being moved in fibrous tissue rather than bone. If it is removed after orthodontic treatment, the scarring may help maintain closure of the diastema.

d)  If the palatal insertion of the fraenum blanches when the lip is lifted, surgery is recommended.

# Answer 4.5

a)  This is a midline supernumerary tooth, known as a mesiodens.

b)  No. Supernumerary teeth usually remain unerupted and are discovered radiographically.

c) The incidence of supernumerary teeth in the permanent dentition is 2% and in the deciduous dentition 1%.

d) Incisors can be displaced from their normal position or fail to erupt due to the presence of a supernumerary. Alternatively, the supernumerary tooth may erupt, aggravating crowding. In general, supernumerary teeth should be removed prior to orthodontic treatment, in order to avoid the risk of potential root resorption of the permanent teeth. However, if they are well away from the teeth to be moved they can be left in place and monitored.

# Answer 4.6

a) The lower left second molar is unerupted, unlike the right second molar which has fully erupted. Asymmetrical eruption patterns should give rise to concern and be investigated, especially if one tooth is fully erupted and the contralateral tooth is not, as seen here.

b) A dental history should reveal if the tooth has been previously extracted, and a radiograph should be used to confirm the presence of the tooth, and its position, or its absence. Surgical removal of any obstruction will be necessary and the patient should be kept under regular review to ensure that the molar erupts. If it fails to erupt spontaneously, then active intervention with fixed orthodontic appliances will be needed.

c) Dentigerous cyst formation around the crown and impaction by the third molar tooth germ are the most common causes of failure of eruption of the second molar. Patients with posterior crowding (i.e. in the molar area) may have a second molar impacted mesially against the first molar. However, this particular case is uncrowded and was found to have a dentigerous cyst associated with the second molar.

# Answer 4.7

a) The bone/periodontal interface demonstrates bone forming activity. The bone is lined by osteoblasts and there is relatively recently formed bone subjacent to these cells.

b) The periodontal ligament has large blood vessels close to the bone. There are fewer vessels adjacent to the cementum. Some have postulated that anti-angiogenesis factors produced by the cementum may be responsible for this.

c) Bone is being laid down here, not resorbed. Therefore the tooth is moving away from this area.

# Answer 4.8

a) This image demonstrates hyalinization, caused by excessive force being applied to the tooth, which compresses the blood vessels in the periodontal ligament.
b) Once the excessive force has been removed, the periodontal ligament will recover. The blood vessels will re-establish themselves and attempts at repair of any cemental damage will be made.
c) Excessive pressure causes pain and also undermining bone resorption (which may slow down tooth movement). The cementum and root are thought to undergo more resorption once they have been exposed to this type of force.

# Answer 4.9

a) The bone at the periodontal interface is being resorbed by multi-nucleated osteoclasts, some of which can be seen lying in their Howship's lacunae.
b) The tooth is moving towards the area of bone resorption, i.e. towards the periodontal ligament/bone interface.
c) The origin of the osteoclast is thought to be fusion of circulating monocytes.

# Removable appliances

## Answer 5.1

a) The fundamental difference between removable and fixed appliances is that removable appliances tip teeth while fixed appliances can move them bodily. Removable appliances tip the tooth about its centre of resistance. This is considered to be the root centroid of single rooted teeth (40% from the root apex), or the trifurcation of multirooted teeth. Removable appliances can also hold blocks of teeth, preventing or allowing selective tooth eruption.

b) The force delivered by a wire spring is controlled by several variables according to the equation:

$$F\alpha \quad \frac{Edr^4}{l^3}$$

where F = force, E = elastic modulus of the wire, d = deflection of the spring on activation, r = wire radius and l = length of the wire. Therefore, the stiffness and thickness of the wire, the degree of activation and its length affect the force delivered by the appliance. The length can be increased by the incorporation of loops. The optimal force is considered to be 25–40 g for single rooted teeth and 40–60 g for multirooted teeth.

c) Removable appliances remain popular in current orthodontic practice for a number of tasks:

   i) tipping teeth, e.g. anterior crossbite correction, overjet reduction, canine retraction, molar distalization, arch expansion, conversion of a class II division 2 to a class II division 1 malocclusion prior to functional appliance therapy

   ii) holding blocks of teeth, e.g. overbite control, space maintenance, retainers

   iii) habit breakers.

d) The advantages of removable appliances over fixed appliances include:
   i) greater effectiveness in achieving certain tooth movements e.g. overbite reduction in a growing patient
   ii) good oral hygiene is easier to maintain
   iii) less chance of root resorption
   iv) minimal chairside time needed for adjustments
   v) straightforward anchorage management if the appliance is worn well.

   The disadvantages of removable appliances are:
   i) success relies on the patient co-operating and wearing the appliance
   ii) only simple tooth movements can be achieved
   iii) only a limited number of tasks can be achieved with one appliance
   iv) they affect speech and increase salivation in the short term
   v) they require an impression for construction, which is never popular
   vi) they require laboratory back-up and time.

# Answer 5.2

a) ARAB stands for:
   i) active components
   iii) retentive components
   iv) anchorage
   v) baseplate.
b) Several designs would work equally well. Here is one possible design:

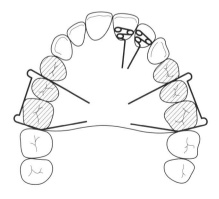

i) double cantilever springs (Z springs) in 0.5 mm stainless steel wire palatal to the upper left central and lateral incisors

ii) double Adams cribs on the upper first and upper second deciduous molars (0.7 mm stainless steel wire)

iii) posterior bite capping

iv) baseplate.

Retention in the middle of the dental arch (i.e. the double crib) is needed because activation of the Z springs anteriorly will displace the appliance downwards. If only the first molars were cribbed the appliance would very easily be displaced.

c) Retention is not necessary after treatment providing the overbite is average or increased, as it will prevent the incisors from relapsing.

# Answer 5.3

a) The anterior component of this appliance is called a Robert's retractor and it is used for reduction of an overjet. It is a high labial bow made from 0.5 mm stainless steel wire supported within 1 mm steel tubing.

b) The Robert's retractor is activated by winding the coil further around using spring forming pliers, so the labial bow moves palatally by 2–3 mm. This can be measured with dividers from the labial bow to a reference point on the baseplate.

c) Other components of removable appliances which can be used to reduce the overjet are:

i) split anterior labial bow in 0.7 mm stainless steel wire

ii) reverse loop Hawley labial bow in 0.7 or 0.8 mm stainless steel wire

iii) open loop Hawley labial bow in 0.7 mm stainless steel wire with additional 0.4 mm wire acting as a strap spring

iv) high labial bow with apron spring

v) elastic band supported on soldered hooks.

d) When fitting the appliance care must be taken to ensure that it is retentive without causing pain. The labial bow must not be overactivated and the acrylic baseplate must be trimmed so that it does not stop desired tooth movement. Therefore, the acrylic must be removed from the palatal aspect of the upper incisors to allow overjet reduction, and the biteplane must be bevelled palatally to enable the palatal soft tissues to settle under the appliance. However, the biteplane must still retain contact with the lower incisors after trimming to enable overbite reduction.

# Answer 5.4

a) This appliance is being used to retract the upper canine, to open space for the missing lateral incisor.

b) Yes. The correct amount of activation for this appliance is seen when the palatal spring lies approximately half way across the canine crown at rest and distal to the canine cusp tip.

c) A buccal canine retractor could be used instead, although this may cause ulceration of the buccal sulcus if it is not carefully constructed.

d) Two possible designs for this appliance are as follows.
First design:

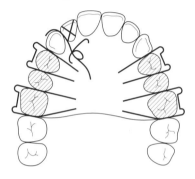

i) palatal canine retractor with palatal guard wire, both in 0.5 mm stainless steel wire, to retract the upper right permanent canine

ii) consider an anterior bite plane if the overbite needs to be reduced

iii) Adams cribs in 0.7 mm stainless steel wire on the first molars and upper first premolars

iv) baseplate.

Second design:

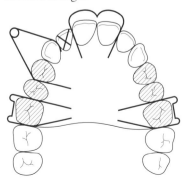

    i)    buccal canine retractor in 0.7 mm stainless steel wire

    ii)   consider an anterior bite plane if the overbite needs to be reduced

    iii)  Adams cribs in 0.7 mm stainless steel wire on the upper first molars

    iv)  Southend clasp in 0.7 mm stainless steel wire to fit the upper central incisors

    v)   baseplate.

e) When fitting the appliance, care must be taken to ensure that it is retentive without causing pain. The springs must not be overactivated, otherwise the baseplate will be displaced and anchorage will be lost. Excessive forces reduce tooth movement by causing the periodontal ligament to become hyalinized. The acrylic baseplate must be trimmed so that it does not stop desired tooth movement, i.e. the acrylic around the canine must be removed to allow distal movement.

# Answer 5.5

a) This appliance is being used to expand the upper arch and to procline the upper lateral incisors out of crossbite.

b) Clinicians vary in their instructions regarding the use of the expansion screw. However, a common instruction is that the screw should be turned by ¼ turn twice a week, i.e. the screw is turned until the next hole becomes visible. This provides expansion at a rate of 0.25 mm per ¼ turn. Some clinicians start with turning the screw ¼ turn once a week.

c) The disadvantage of this method of arch expansion is that it relies totally on patient co-operation, firstly in turning the screw and secondly in turning it in the correct direction. This can be helped by the incorporation of an arrow in the baseplate to show the direction in which the screw should be turned.

d) Other methods of upper arch expansion use:

    i)    a Coffin spring in a removable appliance

    ii)   a quadhelix

    iii)  rapid maxillary expansion

    iv)  expansion with an archwire

    v)   surgical expansion of the maxilla.

e) The posterior bite capping has two functions here. It opens the bite, enabling the upper lateral incisors to procline, and it frees occlusal contacts, enabling the maxillary arch to expand. The patient and parent should be warned that the biteplane will chip in use, but they do not need to return to the surgery unless the appliance breaks.

f) Lifting the T springs gently away from the baseplate activates them. Too much activation will displace the appliance. Alternatively, Z springs in 0.5 mm stainless steel wire could be used. These are slightly more difficult for the patient to seat, but have a longer range of activation than the T springs.

g) The expansion achieved will be the most prone to relapse. The upper lateral incisors should be held in the correct position by the overbite, providing it is sufficiently deep.

h) This appliance is designed as shown:

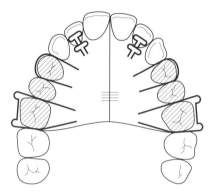

i)    T springs in 0.5 mm stainless wire behind the upper lateral incisors

ii)   midline expansion screw

iii)  Adams cribs in 0.7 mm stainless steel wire on the upper first molars and Jackson's cribs in 0.6 mm stainless steel wire on the upper first deciduous molars

iv)   posterior bite capping

v)    baseplate.

# Answer 5.6

a) The purpose of this appliance is to discourage a digit sucking habit. It is known as a hayrake appliance.

b) The problem with this appliance is that it is removable and the patient can remove it in order to suck their digit! Therefore, success is limited by patient co-operation.

c) The posterior teeth are capped in order to encourage greater eruption of the incisors (which have been intruded by the digit habit) relative to the buccal segment teeth.

d) The tubes soldered to the bridge of the Adams cribs are used for the attachment of a facebow, so that high pull headgear can be fitted to intrude the upper buccal segments, thereby reducing the anterior open bite.

## Answer 5.7

a) Five removable appliance designs:
   i) URA to distalize the upper first molars in conjunction with headgear attached to molar bands

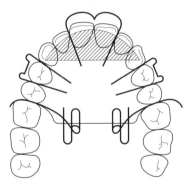

Note: self-guarding palatal finger springs mesial to the upper first molars in 0.6 mm stainless steel wire; flat anterior bite plane; Adams cribs in 0.7 mm stainless steel wire on the upper first premolars; Southend clasp in 0.7 mm stainless steel wire on the upper central incisors; baseplate.

   ii) A clip overbite plane to be used with fixed appliances

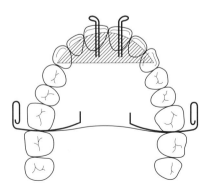

Note: flat anterior bite plane; clip over clasps in 0.7 mm stainless steel wire on the upper first molars; torquing type spurs in 0.5 or 0.6 mm stainless steel wire on the upper central incisors, incisal to the brackets; baseplate.

iii)  A space maintainer for a missing upper left central incisor

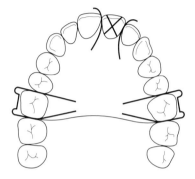

Note: Wire stops mesial to the upper left lateral incisor and upper right central incisor in 0.7 mm soft stainless steel wire; Adams cribs in 0.7 mm stainless steel wire on the upper first molars; baseplate.

iv)  Unilateral screw plate for crossbite correction of the upper right buccal segment

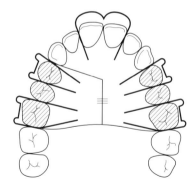

Note: midline expansion screw; Adams cribs in 0.7 mm stainless steel wire on the upper first molars and upper first premolars; Southend clasp in 0.7 mm stainless steel wire on the upper central incisors; posterior bite capping; baseplate, split between the upper right canine and first premolar.

v) Unilateral screw plate for distalization of the upper left buccal segment

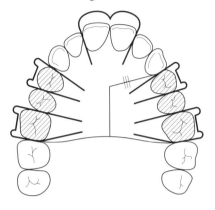

Note: expansion screw orientated anteroposteriorly; Adams cribs in 0.7 mm stainless steel wire on the upper first molars and upper first premolars; Southend clasp in 0.7 mm stainless steel wire on the upper central incisors; posterior bite capping; baseplate, split between the upper left canine and first premolar.

b) In accordance with Newton's third law of motion, all forces have a resultant equivalent force which acts in the opposite direction. Therefore, forces used to distalize teeth will also encourage the unwanted proclination of teeth anterior to the point of force application. This is called anchorage loss. If the overjet increases during treatment, this indicates anchorage loss. Overjet measurement at each visit is a good means of monitoring anchorage management. Anchorage can be controlled by the addition of headgear worn at nights.

## Answer 6.1

a) This appliance is a medium opening activator (MOA) functional appliance.

b) Adams cribs on the upper first molars and the acrylic capping the lower incisors enable the appliance to be retained.

c) Traditionally, a growing patient with a well-aligned class II division 1 malocclusion, a large overjet and deep overbite are ideal for functional appliances. This particular functional appliance is suited to patients with a deep overbite, low maxillary-mandibular planes angle and reduced lower facial height. The lower acrylic extends lingually only in the lower labial segment area and the buccal segments are not capped. These features allow the lower molars to erupt as the overjet is reduced, aiding overbite reduction and increasing the lower facial height.

d) Several limitations affect the use of a MOA. As the appliance is essentially a monobloc, upper arch expansion cannot be carried out at the same time as overjet reduction. Arch expansion must therefore be achieved with an appliance before using the MOA. Unlike the Twin Block appliance, the MOA must be removed for eating, and clear speech is more difficult. This is likely to reduce patient co-operation to part-time wear only. Patients who are predominantly mouth breathers may be assisted with a breathing hole created in the acrylic anteriorly.

## Answer 6.2

a) This is a functional appliance (known as Clark's Twin Block appliance).

b) It is predominantly used to correct large overjets and deep overbites in patients with a class II division 1 malocclusion and normal or increased lower anterior face height. It is particularly useful in the late mixed dentition to reduce the overjet before definitive orthodontic treatment. However, the loss of deciduous teeth during treatment can interfere with the fit of the appliance. Classically, functional appliances are used in class II division 1 cases, where the skeletal discrepancy is mild, crowding is minimal and the dental bases are long. They may also be used in crowded cases and class II division 2 cases, in which the upper incisors can be simultaneously proclined with a spring in the upper removable appliance (URA). Alternatively, a URA to procline and expand the upper arch can be used first.

c)  Functional appliances act by using orofacial muscular forces. Their primary effect is to cause dentoalveolar change, i.e. teeth tip. However, there is some evidence to suggest that condylar repositioning and a minor element of growth modification (maxillary restraint and redirection of mandibular growth) also help to reduce the overjet. Once the overjet has been reduced, the blocks of the Twin Block appliance are trimmed to allow posterior teeth to erupt, thus reducing the overbite.

d)  Twin Blocks have several advantages over other functional appliances. They can be worn 24 hours a day, even during eating. Maxillary expansion with a midline expansion screw can be achieved concurrently with overjet reduction. Speech is normalised more rapidly with the wearing of the appliance 24 hours a day.

e)  Headgear can be attached to soldered extraoral traction (EOT) tubes on the bridges of the Adams cribs or to EOT tubes embedded in the acrylic. The use of EOT will help reduce the overjet and aid restraint of maxillary growth, in the anteroposterior and vertical planes.

## Answer 6.3

a)  This is a Frankel functional appliance. In total, four variants of the Frankel appliance exist: to treat class I cases, class II, class III and cases with anterior open bite or bimaxillary proclination.

b)  Dr Frankel in the former East Germany invented the Frankel appliance. Limited access to fixed appliance components after the Second World War hindered their use, and Dr Frankel created appliances that could more readily be manufactured using available materials. He termed his group of appliances 'function regulators'.

c) Unlike the other functional appliances that use a postured bite to access orofacial muscular forces, the Frankel appliance has carefully positioned buccal and labial acrylic shields. These alter the balance of muscular forces by lifting the soft tissues away from the teeth, enabling them to tip into the space created. Therefore, the correction of the class III malocclusion with this appliance is by dentoalveolar means, not by skeletal modification. The Frankel 2 appliance, used to correct class II malocclusions, has both lingual and labial acrylic pads in the lower labial segment which encourage holding the mandible in a postured position. The buccal shields are extended to fill the buccal sulcus, which Dr Frankel theorised would alter lip behaviour and induce periosteal stretch, therefore stimulating bone formation. There is no evidence to support this theory of skeletal correction.

d) Alternative methods of correcting a developing class III malocclusion include the reverse Twin Block functional appliance, in which the bite blocks displace the mandibular condyles backwards in the glenoid fossae. Chin cup therapy also attempts to limit mandibular development, but studies have shown that its effects are limited to causing the lower incisors to retrocline, without an effect on mandibular growth. Finally, protraction headgear can be used to pull the maxillary dentition forwards. While there is little evidence to show that growth modification can be achieved for skeletal II cases, there is even less evidence to support growth modification in skeletal III cases. The majority of change is achieved by dentoalveolar means and may be transient while active facial growth is continuing. Moderate to severe skeletal III cases may be correctable only with orthognathic surgery.

# Fixed appliances

## Answer 7.1

a)  This fixed appliance is a straightwire fixed appliance with full size A Company brackets.

b)  The fundamental difference between the two appliances is that the straightwire appliance has all the final tooth positions of tip, torque and buccolingual position built into the bracket, by varying the slot angulation, torque and base thickness. Therefore, if the bracket is correctly positioned on the tooth and a maximal dimension rectangular wire is used, the prescribed position should automatically be achieved. Standard edgewise brackets have no such tooth positioning features, hence tooth position is dependent on wire bending. In this picture the wire is not bent (except as an archform), so it is the straightwire appliance.

c)  With the straightwire appliance, final tooth position is dictated by bracket positioning rather than wire bending ability. As the wire remains flat, tooth movement is achieved by sliding mechanics rather than complicated closing loops. Other than modifying archform, wire bending is generally needed only to finish the case to a high standard. Treatment is technically easier and chairside time is much reduced.

d)  The principal components of fixed appliances are those used as means of attachment to the teeth, such as bands and brackets, and active components used to achieve tooth movement, such as wires. Bands are commonly cemented with glass ionomer cement, while brackets are bonded to teeth with composite cement. Glass ionomer cement for bracket bonding has been proposed as a means of reducing decalcification. The bond strength of glass ionomer is approximately half that of composite. Archwires are ligated to the brackets with either elastomeric modules or stainless steel wire. Finally, elastic bands, elastomeric chain and various types of metal coil springs are used for tooth movement. These are commonly attached to hooks on the appliance usually on the bands or archwires.

e) These elastics are attached posteriorly in the mandible, to hooks on the first molar bands, and stretch anteriorly to hooks in the maxillary lateral incisor region. This type of elastic wear is called class II traction.

# Answer 7.2

a) This is the Tip Edge fixed appliance system, which has evolved from the Begg appliance.

b) Unlike the straightwire (and edgewise) fixed appliance systems which move teeth bodily along the archwire to planned positions, the Tip Edge appliance achieves tooth movement by causing the crowns of the teeth to tip along the archwire, often into extraction spaces, before uprighting the roots as a secondary procedure. This method of tooth movement is less demanding on anchorage than bodily tooth movement.

c) Tip Edge treatment is divided into three stages. Stage 1 achieves tooth alignment and reduction of the overbite and overjet. During this stage, only the labial segment teeth and first molars are involved in the appliance. At the beginning of Stage 2 the remaining teeth are incorporated into the appliance and extraction spaces are closed. Stage 3 is primarily concerned with root uprighting and achieving the correct torque. The crowns of the teeth are in the correct positions, but the roots remain tipped. Using rectangular wire and torquing springs (sidewinders) the roots are moved into the correct position.

d) Light class II traction (elastic bands attached between the mandibular molars and the upper lateral incisor/canine region) worn full time, especially during meals, provides much of the mechanical force necessary to achieve tooth movement. Class II traction causes the mandibular molars to extrude and roll lingually, both unwanted effects. This can be limited by tip back bends in the lower archwire, which should also be expanded considerably. Maxillary incisors can also be extruded by class II traction, but this is minimized by tip back bends in the upper archwire which carry the archwire high into the labial sulcus anteriorly. Thus the intrusive effects of the archwire counter the extrusive effect of the elastic.

# Answer 7.3

a) This is a photograph of an upper fixed appliance with ceramic brackets. The upper left permanent canine is unerupted and a steel ligature (laceback) is protecting the archwire in the canine space from occlusal forces.

b) Ceramic brackets have very good aesthetics, although this effect is lessened as the archwire increases in diameter and the elastomeric modules stain. Unfortunately they do have many disadvantages. They increase friction between the bracket and the archwire, reducing the effectiveness of sliding mechanics. Ceramic brackets are harder than enamel and can cause enamel abrasion. For this reason they are not recommended for use on the lower incisors, as the overbite may cause wear to the upper incisal edges. Early types of bracket had excessive bond strength to enamel, causing enamel fractures at debond. Even with modifications to bonding materials and the bracket base, debond is difficult and the brackets may need to be removed with a high speed handpiece. During use tie wings are particularly prone to fracture. Finally, ceramic brackets are expensive.

c) Some brands of bracket incorporate a stainless steel slot to reduce friction, while the bracket base and cement are modified to reduce bond strength to enamel. A careful debonding technique is required. It is helpful to remove excess cement flash from around the bracket base before attempting to remove the bracket.

# Answer 7.4

a) This appliance is a quadhelix.
b) It is used for expansion of maxillary teeth. It can also be activated to achieve molar derotation.
c) The quadhelix should be activated so that when held over the study cast it is expanded relative to the maxillary arch by approximately half a molar tooth width on each side. The palatal arms will then extend along the occlusal surfaces of the teeth. A careful measurement of both the passive and active dimensions should be recorded, so that an indication of the amount of activity remaining in the appliance can be ascertained without the need to remove it from the mouth at each visit. The molar bands are filled with band cement and

the quadhelix is contracted momentarily to its passive dimension whilst cemented in place.

d) The palatal cusp of the first molar tends to drop during expansion and can prop the bite open. This is a problem in cases with reduced overbite. Other problems include tongue irritation. The palatal mucosa may become hyperplastic and the anterior coils may become embedded. The teeth can become excessively mobile. Band cement failure often leads to the appliance becoming dislodged.

e) Alternatives to the quadhelix include an upper removable appliance with midline expansion screw or Coffin spring, rapid maxillary expansion (RME) with a hyrax screw or an expanded upper archwire in a fixed appliance.

# Answer 7.5

a) This appliance is a rapid maxillary expander and aims to open the midpalatal suture.

b) The screw should be turned twice daily, which should provide expansion at a rate of 0.5 mm per day, and the patient should be reviewed about 10 days after fitting.

c) The patient should be warned that a midline diastema will open between their maxillary central incisors.

d) This appliance is used to open the midpalatal suture, across which new bone then forms. Therefore this appliance has an orthopaedic effect, inducing bone formation, and a dentoalveolar effect by displacing teeth buccally. The other expansion appliances have limited orthopaedic effects and work primarily by tipping maxillary buccal segment teeth buccally.

# Answer 7.6

a) An ideal orthodontic archwire should have:
   i)    high strength to withstand occlusal forces
   ii)   low stiffness so that it can be engaged into a bracket
   iii)  a high range of deflection (the distance the wire bends elastically before it is deformed)
   iv)   formability so that it can be bent into hooks
   v)    the ability to accept solder so it can have hooks attached
   vi)   as little friction as possible
   vii)  biocompatibility
   viii) stability in the oral environment
   ix)   low cost.

b) Increasing the cross-section of a wire increases its strength and stiffness, but reduces its range of deflection. Therefore, thicker wires are used as working wires, along which aligned teeth can slide. They are not used for alignment, unless loops are incorporated to alter the length and properties of the wire.

c) Increasing the length of a wire by the incorporation of loops reduces the force applied to the teeth.

# Answer 7.7

a) One of the most recent advances in orthodontic wires is the development of heat activated nickel titanium alloys. On cooling, the wire changes its form from an austenitic form to the martensitic form of nickel titanium. This enables the wire to have superelastic properties, allowing it to engage malpositioned teeth. When the wire reaches mouth temperature the reverse transformation occurs (martensitic to austenitic) and the wire becomes stiff. The advantage of this property is that a rectangular wire can be engaged early in treatment, expressing the bracket torque earlier and possibly reducing the time taken to get into working archwires.

## Answer 8.1

a) This appliance is a lingual arch.

b) Its function is to preserve anchorage in the lower arch, so that all space gained from loss of deciduous teeth or from extractions of permanent teeth can be used as planned. Indications for a lingual arch include:
   i)   severe lower arch crowding requiring all the extraction space for alignment
   ii)  need to preserve space after the loss of deciduous molars
   iii) need to aid correction of a lower centreline shift
   iv)  need to hold space for the eruption or alignment of impacted teeth or of teeth displaced from the arch.

c) Three visits are required to fabricate and fit a lingual arch. Firstly, molar separation with elastomeric separators or brass wire is needed for a week. Following molar band selection, an alginate impression is taken of the lower arch with the bands in situ. The bands are replaced inside the impression (and can be waxed in place) and sent to the laboratory. A stone model is poured and the lingual arch is fabricated. Separation space is maintained with brass wire or elastomeric separators until the following visit. Finally, the appliance is cemented in place.

d) The molar bands may displace within the impression and if not correctly repositioned, this will affect the fit of the appliance.

e) It is possible to fit headgear to the lower arch, but this is even less popular than conventional headgear! A lower removable appliance could be considered but is usually poorly tolerated. A lip bumper attached to the lower molars is a further means of reinforcing lower arch anchorage. Success with these appliances is dependent upon patient cooperation.

# Answer 8.2

a)  This appliance is called headgear and this particular type is the Interlandi headgear.

b)  Headgear use may be considered for both skeletal and dental correction. Vertical and anteroposterior maxillary development can be restrained by headgear use, providing it is worn for an adequate period of time. More commonly headgear is used to control tooth position, e.g. for anchorage support in the upper arch; distalization of upper molars to correct class II buccal segment relationship; overjet reduction; or intrusion of upper buccal segments and/or incisors. The combination of upper molar intrusion and maxillary growth restraint helps to correct a class II skeletal discrepancy. Skeletal change with headgear wear is minor and headgear must be worn over a long period of time (years) to see worthwhile change. Protraction headgear (not shown) is used to bring the maxillary dentition forwards. It may also be used for dental correction of a class III malocclusion or to aid anchorage loss, sometimes required in the management of hypodontia cases.

c)  The component parts of the Interlandi system are a headcap, facebow, elastics and safety strap.

d)  The amount and duration of force application depends on the purpose for which headgear is being worn. For anchorage management, 250 g force applied per side, with wear of 8–10 hours per day is sufficient. However, to achieve tooth movement or growth modification, a force of 500 g per side for 12–14 hours per day is required.

e)  Injury sustained while wearing headgear is rare but has been reported. It includes a penetrating eye injury from a facebow which resulted in blindness. Therefore, safety is very important and headgear should be worn with appropriate safety mechanisms, e.g. a safety strap (pictured) stapled to headcap, snap away headgear and safety locking facebows.

# Answer 8.3

a)  The molar relationship is Angle's class I, but the premolars are slightly class II and the canines are a ½ unit class II.

b)  There are a number of possible explanations for this malocclusion. There is a premolar missing from each arch. This may be due to the developmental absence of second premolars, but it is more likely that the first premolars were removed to relieve crowding. A final class I canine relationship was not achieved, which has limited full correction of the overjet. This poor result may be due to inadequate patient co-operation, resulting in failure to fulfil treatment objectives, or to inadequate anchorage management during active appliance therapy. Alternatively, his dentist may have made a misdiagnosis and incorrectly expected the canines to align spontaneously to class I. Although the explanation is unknown, it is evident that the net result has been anchorage loss. The extraction spaces are closed and no residual space is left to complete alignment of the upper lateral incisor or overjet reduction.

c) The principal problems here are an increased overjet and mild labial segment crowding. Although the canine relationship is ½ unit class II, this does not represent an underlying skeletal problem, but reflects the anchorage loss and crowding. A functional appliance is unsuitable as he has a class I skeletal relationship and class I molar relationship, and the upper incisors do not appear to be proclined. He needs fixed appliance therapy to detail his occlusion. Space is required to align the incisors and reduce the overjet. However, this cannot be created through dental extractions as he has already lost four premolars. Therefore, he needs to be managed with distalization of the upper molars using headgear. In this case, the start molar relationship is class I. Therefore, the final molar relationship will be slightly class III. This will create sufficient space for anterior alignment. Although headgear is not a popular choice, particularly with a possible history of poor co-operation, in this instance it was successful.

# Answer 8.4

a) This is a facemask, commonly known as the Delaire facemask. It is also called protraction headgear.

b) It is used to apply traction to the maxilla. It is useful in class III cases and is gaining increasing popularity in patients with clefts where the maxilla is usually retrusive. It is often helpful in hypodontia cases when the posterior teeth need to be moved mesially and there is concern that the reciprocal effect on the anterior teeth would create a reverse overjet. This is an example of when anchorage needs to be lost rather than enhanced and the facemask can achieve this.

c) The appliance depends completely on patient co-operation. The brow pad and chin cup are uncomfortable to wear, particularly in warm weather when excessive sweating underneath can lead to a skin rash. Cotton linings may help overcome this or, alternatively, perforations in these areas can be introduced. Traction is usually by elastics and if these chafe at the angle of the mouth significant discomfort can arise. Furthermore, saliva passing down the elastics can exacerbate this problem.

d) Elastics attached to hooks on the facemask are used to apply traction either to a removable appliance or fixed appliance. Such traction also keeps the facemask in place on the chin and forehead. The elastics should be attached to the middle of the frame to prevent them chafing at the angle of the mouth.

# 9 Problems

## Answer 9.1

a)  Enamel decalcification has occurred during treatment with fixed appliances. This has progressed to cavitation on the upper right lateral incisor and adjacent canine.

b)  The aetiological factors are the same as for any form of dental caries, i.e. substrate (diet high in sugar), susceptible tooth surfaces and plaque. Carbonated sugar drinks are frequently implicated.

c)  Unfortunately such iatrogenic damage is common. More than 50% of patients have at least one white spot after completion of orthodontic treatment.

d)  Decalcification can be avoided in patients who limit their sugar intake (no carbonated drinks or sweet snacks, including sweet drinks, between meals). Good oral hygiene and fluoride toothpaste are essential. Use of a fluoride mouth rinse at night is also of proven benefit.

e)  Mild decalcification may improve after treatment with subsequent microscopic enamel surface loss. Microabrasion may be applied to moderate surface lesions. Severe cases may need restoration with veneers. Cavities should be managed appropriately, according to their site and severity, and should not be neglected during orthodontic treatment.

## Answer 9.2

a)  This patient has a moderately crowded, mild class III incisor relationship with an intruded upper right central incisor. The intruded incisor is slightly grey in colour compared to the adjacent teeth, suggesting that it is nonvital and space loss has occurred. These signs suggest that this tooth position is a result of an old intrusive traumatic injury occurring subsequent to tooth eruption. Additionally, there is localized

marginal gingivitis.
b) Space has been created to accommodate the central incisor. The dental arches are now in large rectangular steel wires. These are of sufficient rigidity to enable a light, flexible wire (in this instance a nickel titanium wire) to be 'piggybacked' to extrude the intruded tooth. However, the adjacent teeth have become slightly intruded rather than the central incisor becoming extruded, as seen by the loss of the overbite. This suggests that the intruded incisor is ankylosed.
c) Permanent teeth with complete root formation that become traumatically intruded can become rapidly ankylosed, even within a week. Therefore, they should be extruded orthodontically as soon as possible after the injury. Permanent teeth with immature roots have greater chance of spontaneous eruption and do not require immediate treatment. However, they should be kept under close review and treated quickly if signs of devitalization and ankylosis are seen.

# Answer 9.3

a) This is a view of the lingual surfaces of the lower incisors, demonstrating generalised erythema and localized gingival recession.
b) The gingival recession is most likely to be traumatic in origin, compounded by the presence of plaque. In this case, the lingual flange of a medium opening activator functional appliance caused the damage.
c) The source of the trauma must be established and the mucosa must be given opportunity to heal. In this instance the acrylic lingual flange was relieved over the affected area and the patient was advised to leave the appliance out for a few days. Oral hygiene instruction was given.

# Answer 9.4

a) The roots of the upper incisors have undergone resorption during orthodontic treatment.
b) Yes. Root resorption is inevitable to an unpredictable degree during treatment with fixed appliances. However, it rarely compromises the longevity of the teeth.
c) Many risk factors have been associated with this problem:

## Root form

Blunt, pipette shaped or short roots are the most susceptible to root resorption.

## Ectopic canines

Palatally impacted canines are associated with an increased risk of root resorption of the adjacent incisor and premolar teeth. This may be due to increased treatment duration.

## Trauma

Roots already showing signs of resorption due to trauma prior to orthodontic treatment will have increased risk of resorption. Traumatized teeth without root resorption are at no greater risk than non-traumatized teeth.

## Treatment mechanics

Fixed appliances, rectangular wires, class II traction, tooth intrusion and the movement of root apices against cortical bone are all associated with root resorption.

## Age

Patients with complete root formation are at greater risk of root resorption than those with immature root apices.

## Gender

Females are more susceptible to root resorption than males.

## Length of treatment

Longer active treatment is thought to be more damaging than short courses of treatment, although this conclusion is debatable.

## Individual susceptibility

Patients with resorption already will have increased root resorption during orthodontic treatment.

## Systemic problems

Endocrine disturbances such as hyperparathyroidism and hyperthyroidism may increase susceptiblity to root resorption.

d) This problem can be minimized by:
   i) careful history and examination, including radiographs, before treatment can include assessment of the risk factors
   ii) use of light forces and gentle mechanics
   iii) minimizing total length of treatment
   iv) monitoring progress in susceptible patients. Cases with signs of root resorption 6 months into treatment are likely to have severe root resorption at the end of it. Therefore revise treatment aims and consider stopping treatment prematurely
   v) considering the risk/benefit ratio carefully before treatment and warning all patients of the possibility of excessive root resorption occurring.

# Answer 9.5

a) This hyperkeratosis and ulceration of the buccal mucosa is caused by chronic irritation from an overextended archwire.
b) The archwire needs to be shortened and carefully tucked in distally to the last molar band. The patient needs to be given wax when the appliance is first fitted as a temporary solution to irritation from sharp appliance attachments.

# Answer 9.6

a) This is oral candidosis related to wearing an upper removable appliance.
b) This problem needs to be managed by:
   i) the institution of meticulous oral hygiene
   ii) topical antifungal agents
   iii) soaking the appliance in proprietary cleaning solutions
   iv) reassessment of aims of treatment and consideration of alternative approach (e.g. suck down style retainer which does not have palatal coverage) or cessation of treatment.

# Answer 9.7

a) The buccal mucosa bears the imprint of a reverse loop Hawley labial bow, caused by a badly fitting upper removable appliance.
b) The appliance needs to be remade more competently, with careful consideration given to modifying the design so that the wirework is more closely contoured to the teeth.

# Answer 9.8

a) A quadhelix appliance has caused this imprint on the dorsal aspect of the tongue.
b) The quadhelix must be examined to ensure that it contours the palate closely without palatal irritation, and the patient needs simple reassurance that the imprint will resolve when the quadhelix is removed.

# Answer 9.9

a) This is an upper occlusal radiograph of a palatally impacted permanent canine, lying across the apex of the upper incisor. A fixed appliance is attached to the maxillary teeth. A bracket with a chain attachment lies in the vicinity of the impacted canine, having become debonded as traction was applied to the impacted tooth.
b) The aim of treatment was to align the impacted canine. Traction was applied to the canine from the fixed appliance via the chain, but this halted when the bond failed.
c) This problem is difficult to manage, as it now requires a further surgical procedure. The treatment aims should be reassessed and the following considered:
    i)    expose and bond the canine
    ii)   repeat the gold chain procedure
    iii)  remove or transplant the canine.
In this instance the canine tooth was transplanted and splinted with a suck down retainer for two weeks, during which time a pulpectomy with a temporary calcium hydroxide root filling was performed. A permanent root filling was eventually placed.

## Answer 10.1

a) These are removable upper and lower Hawley retainers. The lower has additional labial acrylic to maintain tooth alignment.

b) They are used to maintain tooth position after orthodontic treatment. Teeth will quickly relapse towards their initial position, due to the recoil of the periodontal fibres, if not held in position until fibre remodelling is complete. Individual orthodontists have their preferred regime: full-time wear for 3 months followed by night-time wear for 9 months, missing occasional nights towards the end of the 12 month period, is quite common. Patients can be advised that the longer they wear their retainers, the longer their teeth will stay straight.

c) Unfortunately, relapse to an unpredictable degree is common after orthodontic treatment. Seventy five per cent of cases will have a recurrence of lower incisor crowding. Factors contributing to relapse are: unfavourable soft tissue relationship, such as incompetent lips and tongue thrust; unfavourable skeletal growth; periodontal fibres remaining under tension after treatment; and inappropriate tooth movements which have positioned the teeth out of soft tissue balance.

d) Spaces, such as diastemas, and rotated teeth are particularly susceptible to relapse. Rotated teeth can be overcorrected to aid stability, and the periodontal fibres can be severed electively after derotation (a procedure known as pericision or circumferential fibrotomy). Retention (with fixed or removable retainers) should be long term for those who have unstable features of their malocclusion before treatment. Anterior open bites and deep bites are prone to relapse, as are cases where tooth movement has been performed in order to compensate for severe skeletal discrepancies.

# Answer 10.2

a) This is a fixed retainer.

b) It is used to maintain alignment of the teeth after treatment. Clinical indications for use include spacing (e.g. diastema, periodontal drifting), severely rotated incisors and situations where long-term retention is required and where a removable appliance is undesirable.

c) A common problem in use is that the retainer may become detached from one tooth, which could predispose to tooth decay or relapse if unnoticed. Flossing is difficult but possible with persistence. Bonding a fixed retainer can be time-consuming.

d) An impression of the dentition is taken at the visit prior to debond and a working model constructed. A multistrand wire is shaped, either at the chairside or in the laboratory, to fit to the lingual tooth surfaces in a position where it will be out of occlusion. Following debond, the tooth surfaces are etched, the retainer is held against the teeth and bonded in place with a composite agent. Dental floss, looped around the retainer and through the contact points, or a custom-made acrylic jig are useful aids to hold the retainer in place whilst the composite sets.

e) Alternative options to a fixed retainer include long-term retention with a removable appliance provided that the patient is co-operative. Proprietary fixed retainers consisting of mesh pads and wire are available commercially or are constructed by a dental laboratory. Alternatively, a lingual bar supported by bands on the canines could be used.

f) This patient has two developmentally absent lower incisors.

# Bibliography

Andrews, L.F. (1972). The six keys to normal occlusion. *Am. J. Orthod.*, **62**, 296–309.

Atack, N.E., Turner, S.R., Thomas, P.W.T., Nattrass, C., and Sandy, J.R. (1998). *Postgraduate notes in orthodontics, MSc/MOrth programme*, Bristol University.

Bennett, J.C., and McLaughlin, R.P. (1997). *Orthodontic Management of the Dentition with the Preadjusted Appliance.* Isis Medical Media.

Houston, W.J.B., Stephens C.D., and Tully W.J. (1992). *A Textbook of Orthodontics.* Wright.

McDonald, F., and Ireland, A.J. (1998). *Diagnosis of the Orthodontic Patient.* Oxford University Press.

Mitchell, L. (1998). *An Introduction to Orthodontics.* Oxford University Press.

Mitchell, L., and Mitchell, D.A. (1999). *Oxford Handbook of Clinical Dentistry.* Oxford University Press.

Proffit, W.R. (2000). *Contemporary Orthodontics.* Mosby.

# Index